T0221224

STUDIES IN ANALYTICAL
PSYCHOLOGY

Founded by C. K. Ogden

The International Library of Psychology

ANALYTICAL PSYCHOLOGY
In 12 Volumes

STUDIES IN ANALYTICAL PSYCHOLOGY

GERHARD ADLER

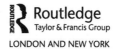

Routledge
Taylor & Francis Group

LONDON AND NEW YORK

First published in 1948 by
Routledge

Reprinted in 1999 by
Routledge
2 Park Square, Milton Park, Abingdon, Oxon, OX14 4RN

Simultaneously published in the USA and Canada by Routledge

711 Third Avenue, New York, NY 10017

Transferred to Digital Printing 2007

Routledge is an imprint of the Taylor & Francis Group, an informa business

First issued in paperback 2013

© 1948 W W Norton & Company Inc

British Library Cataloguing in Publication Data
A CIP catalogue record for this book
is available from the British Library

Studies in Analytical Psychology

ISBN 978-0-415-20938-0 (hbk)
ISBN 978-0-415-86426-8 (pbk)

CONTENTS

ILLUSTRATIONS

I

INTRODUCTION

THESE "Studies in Analytical Psychology" represent a collection of lectures which were given during the ten years from 1936 to 1945. They have all been revised and enlarged, and indeed to a considerable extent rewritten, for the purposes of this book. "A Comparative Study of the Technique of Analytical Psychology" is based on lectures which were given to the post-graduate courses in psychology of the Institute of Medical Psychology (Tavistock Clinic), London, in 1936 and 1937; the "Study of a Dream" is a lecture given to the Medical Section of the British Psychological Society, London, in 1940, and was published (in its original form) in the *British Journal of Medical Psychology*, Vol. XIX, Part I, 1941. "The Ego and the Cycle of Life" was originally delivered in 1939 as a public lecture under the auspices of the Analytical Psychology Club, London, as was also the lecture on "Consciousness and Cure" (delivered in 1938). The latter lecture was published by the Guild of Pastoral Psychology, London, in 1939. "A Psychological Approach to Religion" was given in 1943 at the instigation of the Society of Friends at the Friends' International Centre, London, and again, in a slightly revised form, to the Analytical Psychology Club, London, in 1944. The last paper on "C. G. Jung's Contribution to Modern Consciousness" was written on the occasion of Professor Jung's seventieth birthday for the *British Journal of Medical Psychology* (published in Vol. XX, Part III, 1945) and read to the Analytical Psychology Club, London, in honour of this day on 26th July, 1945. This paper was meant as a birthday gift for Professor Jung, and for this reason I have not felt entitled to change it to any large extent, in contradistinction to all the other papers. As it stands now, it represents more or less an outline and sketch of a research which I hope to be able to produce some day in a much more comprehensive form, giving in detail all the material that could only be hinted at in this essay.

This book is the result of fifteen years of psychotherapeutic practice as an Analytical Psychologist. It has grown out of the almost daily contact between analyst and patient. For this reason I have not tried to give any systematic presentation of Jung's conceptions and of the theory of Analytical Psychology (this, in any case, I have tried to do in a former book: *Die Entdeckung der Seele*, Rascher, Zurich, 1934, which is a systematic survey and comparison of the fundamental conceptions and theories of Analytical Psychology with those developed by Sigmund Freud and Alfred Adler). Every problem discussed in this book has grown out of the common effort of analyst and analysand; and this is valid for the more technical discussions as well as for the more theoretical ones. The latter represent only the effort of the psychotherapist to explain for his own use and that of his patients the experiences of an analysis and to understand the implications of the process of psychological integration.

This fact may serve to explain the order and selection of the essays. The first one is a technical discussion of the method of procedure of Analytical Psychology. It is meant to clarify, both for analysts and for other people interested in psychology, the fundamental differences between the approach of Analytical Psychology and that in particular of Sigmund Freud's Psychoanalysis and to a lesser degree that of Alfred Adler's Individual Psychology. It is also meant to show the limitations of a merely "technical" approach to the "patient," as so often there comes a point where the patient ceases to be a patient and simply reveals the fundamental and commonly valid problems inherent in the psychic growth of every "normal" human being.

The second essay, the "Study of a Dream," is meant to exemplify a fundamental conception of Analytical Psychology, that of the *collective unconscious* and the *archetypes,* and to show both its practical implications and its application in actual treatment.

The conception of the collective unconscious, namely of a common substratum of general psychic inheritance which cannot be explained by personal experience—and of the archetypes, that is: of the images in which the collective unconscious manifests itself—is indispensable for an understanding of the approach of Analytical Psychology, both in its practical and its theoretical aspects. The collective unconscious is, as Jung has said, "the all-controlling deposit of ancestral experience from untold millions of years, the echo of prehistoric world-events to which each century adds an infinitesimally small amount of variation and differentiation"; it is "a sort of timeless world-image."[1] Its scope is much larger than that of the personal psyche—including both the personal conscious and the personal unconscious (i.e. the unconscious contents which have been acquired during the personal existence of the individual)—and it has therefore energies at its disposal which are more potent than those of the personal psyche. Although the conception of the collective unconscious is the red thread running through the whole book, this particular essay may help the reader to understand its practical therapeutic value more clearly.

The third essay on "The Ego and the Cycle of Life" illustrates the different psychological problems inherent in different phases of life. It shows how the process of psychic growth and maturation, that is the process of integration and individuation, presents the individual with widely different situations and tasks according to the particular point he has reached in life. While the process of individuation is illustrated here from the practical point of view, the next essay on "Consciousness and Cure" approaches the same problem from the theoretical, and indeed from a philosophical, angle. Starting with the concrete problem presented by the two dreams of a patient, an attempt is made to understand the psychological force that is at work when a cure is achieved. This force is defined as an unconscious, *a priori* image of psychic "wholeness" in the psyche which works towards its own realiza-

[1] Jung, *Contributions to Analytical Psychology*, Kegan Paul, London, 1928, p. 162.

tion and actualization. Although this enquiry is theoretical, it has nevertheless considerable practical implications, as analyst as well as analysand are constantly confronted with the problem of how a cure is effected, and an understanding of the forces at work is bound to have repercussions on the practical work.

In the fifth essay an attempt is made to define the point of view of Analytical Psychology with regard to religion. This again may seem to be a more or less theoretical discussion, but in point of fact it is highly practical as so many of the conflicts and problems of our patients reveal themselves as problems of a spiritual and, in the widest sense of the word, religious crisis. The term "religious" is taken to comprise the genuine and irreducible impulse in man which forces him to find an answer to the question of the spiritual meaning and significance of his life. It has to be said that psychology in its merely analytical and reductive aspects— first and foremost psychoanalysis—has only too often failed to recognize and face the reality of this problem. Instead of realizing the genuineness and poignancy of the religious urge in man, a psychology that misunderstood its own scope and task, and tried to limit the psyche of man to merely personal and, in the narrow sense of the word, instinctual drives, has attempted to reduce religion to a "mechanism of escape." The genuine and irreducible spiritual and religious impulse has thus been reduced to a particular aspect of the "family novel," and God to an inflated image of the personal father.[1]

[1] Jung has pointed to the important fact that Freud's "super-ego" is a projection of the unconscious image of the "self." The collective moral consciousness—the "conscience"—which the super-ego represents is according to Freud derived from the child's fear of the parents; it is the representative of our relationship to the parents, and as such "the heir of the Oedipus-complex." (Cf. Freud, *The Ego and the Id*, Hogarth Press, London, 1927, p. 47f.). This point of view overlooks the fact that our "conscience," our inner moral and ethical laws, our inner voice, or whatever else one may like to call these formative forces, are due to *a priori* conditions of the human psyche which are not acquired during our personal existence, but only become manifest in it. They are, in other words, manifestations of the non-ego, or self. As long as we are still unconscious of the self, it appears projected into the environment (e.g. the parents). With the growing integration of the self the projection is withdrawn, and the "moral law" is experienced as an *a priori* condition of our psyche. (Cf. Jung, *Das Wandlungssymbol in der Messe*, in: *Eranos-Jahrbuch* 1940–1941, Zurich 1942, p. 136ff.)

This has produced an unfortunate situation in that people, although they are aware of their deep spiritual problems and needs, have been discouraged from connecting their most urgent question with psychology and thus do not expect an answer from it. Through psychology being thus wrongly identified with the one-sided approach of the reductive schools, it has come to be regarded as mere psychopathology. Psychoanalysis and other merely reductive schools of modern psychology have focused too exclusively on the pathological manifestations of the psyche; and thus they have cornered man in his neurosis. It seems most important to widen the meaning of "therapy" through the realization that psychotherapy is not just a "mental cure" but a much more comprehensive way to self-knowledge. This naturally includes the spiritual side of man just as much as his biological side; as a matter of fact, the spiritual side has to be accepted as the really decisive manifestation—because the characteristically human one—of the psychic process. Only if people realize that psychology does not attempt to reduce their spiritual problems to nothing but sex or power or any other drive, but accepts these as the inevitable and creative effort to find an answer to the meaning of their lives, can psychology fulfil its proper function of dealing with the totality of human life.

In this sense the last essay on "C. G. Jung's Contribution to Modern Consciousness" tries to define the historical situation in which psychology finds itself. It is an attempt to trace the psychological images active in the formation of the modern mind; in other words it deals with the archetypal aspect of this historical development. It tries to show the particular position of Analytical Psychology in modern consciousness: how through the work of C. G. Jung the way has been prepared for a synthesis between the rational and scientific side of Western man on the one hand and his irrational and religious side on the other. The "masculine" and "feminine" aspects are discussed in their archetypal significance, leading to a possible and indeed necessary *conjunctio* of the two which would mean a true totality of man. It has become only too obvious in our days, overshadowed as they are by the fear of the atomic bomb, how urgent the need is for man's scientific and rationalistic side to be balanced by a new sense of religious and relational values. The loss of the latter was largely due to the impact of the scientific-rationalistic tendencies in man, which in their youthfulness tended to deny the right of any other approach, which was derisively termed "unscientific."[1] The important development in psychology inaugurated by C. G. Jung has been that in applying the scientific attitude to man's own nature, he discovered in the human psyche the super-personal images of the collective unconscious, the archetypes, as "the *a priori* determining constituents of all experience."[2] They are "involved in the peculiarities of the living organism itself, and are therefore immediate expressions of life whose nature cannot be further explained."[3] The discovery of the archetypes has shown that a purely rationalistic and personalistic conception of the human psyche is thoroughly unsatisfactory and artificial, for they transcend both the personal experience and the limitations of intellect. Jung proved for instance the presence of an archetype of the Deity in the human psyche as an *a priori* condition of irrational and super-personal experience.

This archetype of the Deity in the human psyche Jung has termed the "self." It is the immanent goal of individuation and at the same time it is the power which drives man towards the achievement of his integrated individuality. This goal can only be attained by an ever-increasing consciousness which, through constant application and a corresponding awareness of the psychic process, tries to find the way back to its own sources. It is not enough for modern man simply to believe what other people before him have believed and because they have believed it,

[1] This must not be misunderstood as a rejection or criticism of science as such, but only of its exaggerated claims. Jung has formulated this point of view clearly when he says: "Science is the best tool of the western mind, and with it more doors can be opened than with bare hands. Thus it is part and parcel of our understanding and only clouds our insight when it lays claim to being the one and only way of comprehending." (*The Secret of the Golden Flower*, Kegan Paul, London, 1931, p. 78.)

[2] Jung, *Contributions to Analytical Psychology*, p. 276.

[3] Jung, *Two Essays on Analytical Psychology*, Baillière, London, 1928, note 1 to p. 71.

without questioning and doubting; he wants and needs immediate knowledge which can be attained only through personal experience produced by unprejudiced enquiry.

This puts quite a new responsibility on human consciousness. If the discovery of the archetypes as the *a priori* determining constituents of all experience means that the real lead is with the unconscious, it also means, on the other hand, that the individual, through his conscious mind, has to experience, to choose and to decide for himself. "To be conscious" becomes thus the maxim and the measure of psychological maturity and achievement. This state of "being conscious," however, needs a clear definition. The meaning of the word "conscious" as given by the *Shorter Oxford English Dictionary* is to be "aware of what one is doing or intending to do." Such an awareness is only possible if one is sufficiently familiar with one's own psychology, which presupposes a more or less clear perception and assessment of one's own motives and conditionings. The fact, however, is that this knowledge is one of the most difficult things to attain. Although we seem most of the time to act as quite "sensible" human beings, we are nevertheless driven to a large extent by "unconscious" motivations, i.e. by impulses of which we are not aware; and although we may appear as more or less clearly defined personalities, we are nevertheless unconsciously identified with circumstances or other people, and we are thus not at all independent "individuals."

To be an individual, to possess individuality, implies being distinct from others; "the psychological individual is characterized by its peculiar, and in certain respects, unique psychology."[1] Although everybody possesses such individuality *in potentia*, in actual fact it needs awareness of one's own specific characteristics, one's own "uniqueness," before the individuality becomes established. As long as I am not conscious of my own psychology, I am bound to "project" it on to other people or things. The process of projection is one of the fundamental psychic mechanisms. It is singularly noticeable in the psychology of primitives (and of

[1] Jung: *Psychological Types*, Kegan Paul, London, 1923, p. 560.

children) where, for example, it is the foundation of the belief in spirits; psychic facts such as fears or desires are not experienced by primitive man as part of his own psyche but projected on to his surroundings and objectified as demons or evil spirits. Thus the primitive (and the child) is to a large extent identified with his environment because this contains considerable parts of his own psychology.

What is valid for primitive man is also valid to a lesser degree for civilized man as long as he is still "unconscious" of the contents of his own psyche. On the one hand projection is a first and inevitable step towards consciousness, because everything in myself of which I am unconscious is projected, and so it is through projection that I am first confronted with an inner psychic content. On the other hand, as long as the next step is not taken, as long as the projection is not withdrawn from the object into the subject, the state of projection represents a danger to the psychic balance and stability as it is a state in which man's psyche is split up into many parts and more or less tied to his environment. As long, for instance, as I am unconscious of my own "shadow," namely the "dark" and inferior side of my own psychology, I am bound to project it on to somebody else, and the same is true for the potential "wholeness" of my own psyche, in which case somebody else may be invested by me with qualities of superhuman or quasi-magical powers. In every case of projection a kind of fascination results, since I am tied to the parts of my own psychology which I have projected; in the case of the shadow-projection I am tied to the other person in hatred, in the case of the "saviour"-projection I am tied to the other person in blind and uncritical adoration. For the first case the obsession of the Nazis with the Jews presents a tragic example, for the second the almost divine power with which they invested the "Führer." To go back a few centuries, the trials of witches present another convincing example both of the shadow- and "anima"-projection; in this case men projected their own powerful primitive and therefore dreaded feminine side into the witch and women had found unconsciously the scapegoat for their own "dark" side.

In other words, as long as I am "unconscious," as long as I "project," I am identified with other people or things, be it in "hatred" or "love"; I live in a state of *"participation mystique"* with somebody or something else. This is, of course, a state in which no true individuality exists. Such individuality can only develop if I become conscious of my own psychology and learn to assimilate my unconscious contents. The assimilation of the contents of the personal unconscious is always the first step towards complete integration. These contents are largely due to "repressions,"[1] as they represent those desires, fears or other tendencies of my psyche which are incompatible with my ego-personality, whether it be because they are too infantile or too unpleasant or for some other reason. The integration of the personal unconscious is therefore always a difficult process and asks for a considerable amount of moral courage. Without it, however, the integration of the progressive and constructive contents of the collective unconscious is impossible.

"To be conscious" then is the first and foremost demand of psychological integration. It means to withdraw one's projections and to become "de-identified." To become conscious is therefore not an intellectual act, but implies an emotional quality of realization which involves the whole of the personality. Somebody may be intellectually aware of his problems, he may even be able to give a more or less complete psychological history of his neurosis, and still he will not be cured as long as the emotional realization which commits his whole personality has not taken place. Genuine consciousness means a constant responsibility towards a centre which has been realized and accepted as "true"; to be "unconscious" means to be caught in the trap of identifications and ulterior motives.

In order to avoid misunderstandings one more word must be added with regard to the unfortunately equivocal meaning of the terms "conscious" and "unconscious." It has been said above

---

[1]Jung defines the personal unconscious as all the "acquisitions of the personal existence—hence the forgotten, the repressed, the subliminally perceived, thought, and felt" matter of every kind. (*Psychological Types*, pp. 615–16.)

that in the integrated personality the lead lies with the unconscious whereas the conscious mind has to choose and to decide. Obviously the term "unconscious" has here a different meaning from that which it has in the statement that "to be unconscious means to be caught in the trap of identifications." In the first statement the word "unconscious" has a positive, progressive connotation, in the second case a negative, regressive one. This latter could be best described as a state of "unconsciousness," which has to be distinguished from "the unconscious" as the foundation of psychic life to which the first statement refers. The unconscious psyche, in Jung's sense, is the matrix of the conscious psyche; it is far older and far more comprehensive than the latter. The conscious psyche—of which the ego is the representative—could be compared to the top of a pyramid, and it is clear that the top would be in an unenviable position if the broad basis underneath were taken away. Through being so much older and more comprehensive than the conscious psyche, the unconscious psyche contains images and potential realizations full of instinctive wisdom, and it is these that the conscious psyche must learn to perceive and to integrate. In this sense the term "the unconscious"—or more precisely: the collective unconscious, or nonego—connotes the eternal matrix and nourishing source of the conscious psyche. On the other hand, Jung defines the conscious mind as "the function or activity which maintains the relation of the psychic contents with the ego."[1] In this sense "to be conscious" is the indispensable presupposition for psychic integration, and "to be unconscious" means to be unaware of psychic contents, and therefore to be at their mercy.

From what has been said it is apparent that the term "conscious" also has a double meaning. If on the one hand "to be conscious" is the condition of psychic integration and "consciousness" the achievement of it, on the other hand it must not be forgotten that the "conscious psyche" is only a part, and by far the smaller one, of the whole psyche. The conscious mind is not identical with the psyche, in as far as the psyche represents the

[1]Jung, *Psychological Types*, p. 536.

totality of *all* psychic contents, conscious as well as unconscious ones. Where a person identifies his psychic contents with the conscious psyche alone, he has more or less cut himself off from the basis and root of his consciousness, and is trying to perform the proverbially impossible operation of cutting off the branch on which he sits. Where the conscious psyche has thus become alienated from its foundation, it necessarily works in an unbalanced and therefore, in the long run, destructive way. It is thus only in their mutual relationship that the value and function of both the unconscious and the conscious psyche can be understood. Where a person is "too conscious" only, he is, to put it in a paradoxical way, in reality unconscious of the unconscious; i.e. the connection with the instincts and the eternal foundations of realization has been lost, and the way back and down into the unconscious has to be opened up again. When, on the other hand, a person is living too much in the unconscious, when he is too much identified with the collective images, the conscious side— the ego—has to be developed. (This problem is dealt with in particular in the essay on "The Ego and the Cycle of Life.") Generally speaking the problem of realizing the dependence upon and the creative value of the unconscious—particularly in its deeper impersonal collective layer—has become the foremost problem of Western man with his increasing over-differentiation of the conscious mind and his insistence on its omnipotence. Eastern civilization hardly knows of an individual ego in our Western sense. The conscious mind of Western man seems to be the only one which has separated itself from nature. For this very reason it is the particular task of the West to integrate the *inner* nature, that is the collective unconscious.

Strictly speaking, one should therefore distinguish between "the conscious mind" and "consciousness." In the strict sense the "conscious mind" is that limited part of the psyche which both opposes the unconscious psyche and completes it so that the two make up the totality of the psyche. "Consciousness" on the other hand, is the result of becoming conscious of a smaller or greater part of the whole psychic situation, comprising both the unconscious and the conscious psyche; it has thus a wider meaning than the term "the conscious mind" as it is the result of the application of the latter to the unconscious background of the psychic situation. "To become conscious" in the constructive sense of the word means to integrate and assimilate more and more of the contents of the unconscious without ever losing sight of the fundamental interdependence of the unconscious and the conscious psyche, resulting in a more or less complete "consciousness." In other words: the integration of the (collective) unconscious gradually leads to a stronger and more comprehensive consciousness. "Conscious assimilation of unconscious contents" means thus "a mutual interpenetration of conscious and unconscious contents, and not—as is too commonly thought—a one-sided valuation, interpretation and deformation of unconscious contents by the conscious mind."[1] A decisive conception of Analytical Psychology is that of the psyche as a "self-regulating system" which means that "the unconscious processes . . . contain all those elements that are necessary for the self-regulation of the total psyche."[2] Where this process of self-regulation is properly understood, where the conscious and the unconscious psyche thus work together in a constructive way, the aim of the individuated and integrated personality can be achieved. This book is an attempt to describe this fundamental idea of the psyche as a self-regulating system aiming at the individuation and integration of the personality.

[1]Jung, *Modern Man in Search of a Soul*, Kegan Paul, London, 1933, p. 18f.
[2]Jung, *Two Essays on Analytical Psychology*, p. 189.

ACKNOWLEDGMENTS

I SHALL not attempt to say what this book owes to Professor Jung. What I owe not only to his writings, but even more to personal contact with him, becomes more and more apparent to me every day. Next to him I want to thank Miss Toni Wolff, to whose unfailing friendship and critical advice I am more indebted than words can express.

Miss Monica Curtis' patient and understanding revision of the English text has been a great help to me throughout the final composition of this book. I should also like to thank Miss Lorel Goodfellow for her beautiful work in translating the earlier essays in their original form, and I feel much indebted to the friends who have given me helpful advice in correcting the essays for print. And lastly I would not forget my patients, who gave me their confidence, and with it the courage and the stimulus to present the experiences of our common work in this form. There is no greater reward for the psychotherapist than the experience of his daily work.

I I

A COMPARATIVE STUDY OF
THE TECHNIQUE OF ANALYTICAL
PSYCHOLOGY

IN ANY attempt to discuss the technique of Analytical Psychology within a comparatively limited compass, certain important reservations must be made at the outset. In the first place, the technique of Analytical Psychology is so large a subject that it would not be possible to give a comprehensive account of it; what is aimed at is therefore a kind of general survey, with particular emphasis on the differences between Analytical Psychology and other schools of modern psychotherapy, especially that of Sigmund Freud. The idea of such a survey can only be to give an outline of the general principles of analytical treatment. This necessarily involves a certain amount of theoretical discussion. As, however, this theoretical discussion will be illustrated by material obtained from actual psychotherapeutic treatment, it may be hoped that the general line of treatment will emerge clearly.

A second limitation lies in the fact that Analytical Psychology is only one among several schools of modern psychotherapy, all of which place the concept of the unconscious in the very centre of their field of vision. From this it follows that the technique of Analytical Psychology coincides with the techniques of other methods of modern psychotherapy, as for example that based on the theories of psychoanalysis, in a number of points where their basic conceptions are the same. This means that the methods of Analytical Psychology in practice are sometimes less unlike those of other schools than might be supposed.

The third and most important limitation is due to the fact that one of the main differences between Analytical Psychology and other schools lies in the undogmatic approach of Analytical Psychology to each individual case. The basic presupposition from which Analytical Psychology starts is that each patient has his own particular and "personal" psychology, necessitating an approach which varies with each individual case. As Jung has said "The investigation of truth begins with each case anew, because any living truth is individual and not to be derived from any previously established formula. Each individual is an experiment of everchanging life, and an attempt at a new solution or new adaptation."[1] Such a conception must obviously involve a considerable limitation on general technique, since the whole point of a technique is to provide certain universally applicable rules. This may be deplored in so far as value is traditionally attached to general principles; but, on the other hand, the willingness and capacity of the psychotherapist to approach each individual case without hard-and-fast theories is the touchstone of whether he is suitable to be a psychotherapist. For just as every scientist who undertakes a series of experiments has to forget all his preconceived theories and to focus his attention solely on the unprejudiced observation of facts *as they happen,* so psychologists have to approach each new patient—each new "experiment of life"—without any preconceived ideas. Theories are nothing but an *a posteriori* attempt to give an order to certain natural events in such a way as to present the scientist with a new question from which to start on a new enquiry. Thus each patient has to be a new question-mark to the psychotherapist, and his theoretical deduction can be nothing more than an attempt after the event to understand the case better.

Moreover, according to the particular psychological situation in which a human being is placed, different psychological needs arise. Thus the method of psychotherapy required in the case of a man who has achieved adaptation to external reality and its necessities may be different from the method suitable for one who lives in an inner world of ideas, but remains unadapted to the

[1]Jung: *Contributions to Analytical Psychology,* p. 349.

external world. Different phases of life, different types of personality, different needs, require different approaches. Elasticity and adaptability to the case in hand are of cardinal importance, for any dogmatic conception which neglects these different psychological constellations may cause the most serious damage to the patient's psychological development. For all these reasons it is only possible to try to indicate the general lines of treatment, certain guiding principles as it were, which Analytical Psychologists adopt towards their patients, without attempting to erect them into any hard-and-fast technique or system of rules.

When a patient comes for treatment, it is obviously necessary to start by clearing the field with regard to certain very general matters which are so universal that they represent common ground to every psychotherapist to whatever school he may belong. Since they also apply to the methods of treatment of Analytical Psychology, they must be mentioned in order to give a more complete picture, although in view of their universality they can be dealt with briefly. One of the first questions which a new patient asks his analyst is how long the treatment is likely to take. This question is as inevitable as it is justifiable, and one which every analyst expects and none can answer. There is only one rule to observe: never, in order to encourage a patient to begin treatment, hold out the hope that the time required will be short. The best way out of this insoluble dilemma, and at least a partial answer, is to suggest that the patient should begin with a trial analysis lasting say four weeks. The advantages of this are twofold: first of all, it will enable a psychotherapist of any experience to form some kind of picture of the case and its attendant difficulties, and to make some guess at the probable duration of treatment; secondly, and even more important, he will discover whether the particular case is or is not suitable for analysis at all. In this way the patient can be saved the dangerous disappointment of an unsuccessful analysis. Even after such a trial analysis it will be impossible to give any exact indication of the length of treatment, but only its probable duration. As a rule one should never reckon in weeks, but rather in periods of six months. Experience shows that the *minimum* time (leaving out of account exceptional cases where the symptoms are quite superficial) required for any fundamental change is from six months to a year. It is obvious that the mention of such a lengthy period of time is likely to give the patient a shock, but an analysis makes such tremendous demands on a patient and requires so many sacrifices, both spiritual and material, that his willingness to submit to such a long and expensive treatment is often the touchstone of his capacity to undergo an analysis at all. It should be made clear to the patient right from the beginning that analysis is not a kind of magical charm which will lift him out of his problems in a second, but that it represents a thorough re-orientation, which demands the willing application of his whole personality. Only if he is prepared to accept this fact, and the expenditure of time, energy and money which it involves, will he be able to receive the full benefit of a true depth-analysis. Besides, any under-estimate of the length of time required will in the course of treatment inevitably be used against the analysis, since it provides the patient with a superb cloak to mask his latent resistance to the analysis and the analyst. Moreover, since he has actually been misled by the psychotherapist, the apparent justification which is thus given to his resistance may well make it assume dangerous proportions.

Another question is that of fees. Unfortunately a psychological analysis is a somewhat expensive business; and often enough, it is quite impossible for the patient to produce the necessary financial resources. Regular payments should nevertheless be insisted on, even with financially distressed patients. The payment, even though small, should stand at least as a symbol; for money, apart from its very concrete significance, carries with it quite definitely the symbolical value of an expenditure of energy; and the payment of money therefore symbolically represents the recognition that energy is to be expended. Quite apart from the point of view of the psychotherapist, for whom every gratuitous treatment means an almost unendurable sacrifice of time and energy —a sacrifice which in the last resort must react unfavourably on his own capacity for work—the situation of the patient has to be considered from the psychological angle. From the patient's point of view, a gratuitous analysis is thoroughly unsound; the very fact that it is gratuitous constitutes an almost insuperable difficulty. Thus a young man, for instance, may easily be driven into the most determined resistance, for owing to the father transference to the analyst, he will react violently against the feelings of gratitude which are forced upon him if the treatment is gratis. Similarly, in the case of a male psychotherapist, free treatment may make it almost impossible for a woman patient to resolve a transference and vice versa. Again, there may be the case of the patient who finds it too difficult to tell the psychotherapist about his negative emotions because "the analyst has been so kind to him"—a splendid cloak for resistances. If, on the other hand, the patient pays even a small amount—but it should always be an amount that represents a substantial value to him—he can feel himself to be a more equal partner in the analytical situation. Obviously there are cases in which free treatment is unavoidable, but too great care cannot be exercised in their choice, and one should never lose sight of the fact that free treatment itself always creates a specific and serious additional difficulty. This fact may well be deplored; but its realization is unavoidable. We must be careful that as psychotherapists we are not ourselves influenced by any money complex of our own, and that we do not react in an unconscious and therefore unadapted manner.

As regards the frequency of treatment, it is usual to start with two to three hours a week. In certain cases of exceptional gravity it is sometimes desirable and occasionally necessary to increase this number. If there are fewer than two weekly interviews, the intervals are too long and the effect of the analysis suffers. Besides, decreasing the number of weekly interviews does not save the patient anything in the long run, since it merely prolongs the analysis. On the other hand, it is usual not to see patients more than two or three times weekly, because experience has shown that the rhythmical change between the analytical interview and a period of assimilation is most valuable. The unconscious finds time to react to the analytical discussion, and the normal flow of life is not broken up. For a similar reason, it is recommended that the patient should be accustomed to definite weekly times, as his unconscious then adjusts itself to a certain rhythm. With the passage of time, that is with the patient's growing independence and towards the end of the analysis, these intervals are increased till the interviews take place only once a week or even less frequently. This latter point will be discussed later.

One of the fundamentals of psychotherapy is the *external* relationship of psychotherapist and patient. This involves important questions of principle, and here Analytical Psychology differs in one vital respect from the attitude adopted by psychoanalysis. The Freudian psychoanalyst gets his patients to lie down while he takes up a position behind them and outside their line of vision. We prefer to sit opposite to them and face to face. There are occasions on which I may get patients to lie down, for instance if they are very strung up and tense and I want them to relax, but even so I sit down opposite to them and in full view. From the technical point of view, the main objections to the patient's lying down while the analyst remains invisible in the background are these: (1) The passive rôle of the patient is overemphasized "as if an operation were being performed on him." (2) It makes it easier for the patient to shut himself off in an artificial vacuum, and (3) it therefore makes it more difficult for him to bridge the gap which separates him from the analyst, enabling him to relegate the experiences which he undergoes during analysis to an unreal world entirely cut off from every-day life. On the other hand, to sit face to face immediately produces a more natural and more human situation. It makes it much more difficult for the patient to use the analyst as a lay figure on which to hang his projections without testing what degree of reality they possess. It minimizes the distance between them and puts them into immediate human contact.[1]

[1]Another factor in this situation is the different emphasis on "free associations" and dream-interpretation (cf. p. 44ff.). Where, as in the psychoanalytical method, the main accent is on free associations, that is on an attitude in which the patient is more or less kept to himself, lying down without seeing the analyst is at least more suitable than where dream-interpretation with its much more active exchange between patient and analyst forms the main element of analysis, as it does in the procedure of Analytical Psychology.

This technical difference in the external position expresses at the same time a fundamental difference in the whole attitude to the patient. If you sit behind your patients, without coming into view, you assume symbolically a completely unassailable position, that of a superior being over against whom the patient's own personality and worth sink into nothingness; you corner the patient in his neurosis. To sit face to face, on the other hand, is to admit symbolically that the patient is indeed in certain respects ill and in need of treatment, but that nevertheless he himself still exists as an independent entity. It is illuminating that in psychoanalysis the conception of a man's character as a unique, individual, psychic constellation, plays scarcely any part, and that all the emphasis is laid on fundamental instincts common to all men. But this view disregards precisely that aspect of any given personality which is unique and creative. That aspect is still expressed in the neurosis, albeit in a formless and indirect way. In our opinion, a neurosis conceals certain positive and creative values, since every neurosis is really an attempt, although an unsuccessful one, to compensate for that very one-sidedness of the conscious attitude which led to the neurosis; for the conscious mind never contains all the possibilities of any individual. In this sense every neurosis is really an unconscious attempt at a new adaptation. If, however, one approaches every neurotic patient with a cut-and-dried set of definite dogmatic preconceptions, such as that every neurosis is nothing but a failure in sexual adaptation or an unsuccessful expression of the will to power, one fails at the very outset to come to grips with his unique individual personality.

The Jungian conception of the individual and positive values inherent in every neurosis explains the difference between the conception of transference in Analytical Psychology and in psychoanalysis. To the latter, transference must represent a sexual phenomenon because every psychic disturbance is understood to conceal an infantile sexual problem, as the unconscious merely consists of repressed sexual tendencies. In the view of Analytical Psychology, however, transference represents the projection on to the psychotherapist of the patient's unconscious, which by no means contains nothing but sexual wishes. It is a general rule that every unknown content of our unconscious is projected on to other human beings or even objects. This is especially obvious in the psychology of primitive races. Thus, a primitive man projects his emotions into his surroundings. These therefore appear to him charged with spiritual power, so-called mana, which is really derived from the energy of his own unconscious. A similar mechanism is at work wherever we are unaware of our psychic contents. Analytical Psychology therefore looks on transference as the mechanism by which the patient projects on to the person of the analyst those aspects of his life which are hidden in his unconscious. Obviously the transference often enough assumes a definite erotic tinge, more especially in the case of patients with strongly marked autoerotic and narcissistic tendencies. In such cases the unconscious compensates for a former onesidedness by expressing the patient's need—and capacity—for entering into human relationships, a need which he had hitherto repressed or neglected. The patient must be helped to realize his undeveloped potentialities in this direction by facing the problem of his relationship to the psychotherapist. If, on the other hand, the analyst assumes the rôle of a magician or medicine-man in the eyes of an over-developed rationalist, this is by no means a sexual projection on his part, nor even necessarily a father projection, but it does express the non-rational energies of his psyche which such a pronounced rationalist would be the last to acknowledge.

These examples show that Analytical Psychology does not consider transference merely from the point of view of repressed infantile sexuality, but takes a view of its mechanism which differs fundamentally from that of psychoanalysis. The psychoanalyst considers transference his main therapeutic agency, inasmuch and in so far as in this way, by means of the "reproduction-urge," the repressed contents of the unconscious are re-enacted on the person of the analyst, and are thus once more brought into consciousness.

On the other hand, Analytical Psychology regards this process as the projection of psychic contents which are lost to consciousness, e.g. by repression, in which case they belong to the layer of the "personal unconscious," or, more important, which are still subliminal, in which case they are mainly of an archetypal character. Very often there is hidden underneath the projection of contents belonging to the personal unconscious a deeper level of archetypal contents, and analysis reveals the preliminary character of the former. Projections are almost unavoidable at the beginning of an analysis; but dreams may fulfil the same function as transference, since they furnish all the material required in the analysis of the unconscious. In actual fact, both dreams and projections often go together.

We thus do not look on transference as a mechanism for re-experiencing repressed infantile sexual impulses, but as a phenomenon by means of which the patient becomes aware of psychic functions that have been lacking in his conscious life. Transference in this sense is the constellation of the unconscious and thereby an attempt at compensation for the onesidedness of the patient's personality. Transference may help to activate contents of the unconscious which are necessary for the future development of the psyche. This is in particular the case where archetypal images are projected. Therefore it often conceals a source of energy which the patient has not yet found inside himself. Only when he discovers this energy in his own unconscious and integrates it into consciousness can the transference be "dissolved."

In this sense the transference, besides constellating unconscious contents, can be understood to fulfil a particular function; it acts as a kind of magic circle inside which the patient is held until the meaning of the psychological situation has been properly understood. Not before the integration of the particular psychic content has been achieved, does the magic circle open. It is as if the patient's inmost and deepest need becomes manifest in this force which holds him down to the analysis through the power of the transference situation.

Transference is really only one particular case of the wider phenomenon of projection; that is, we talk of transference if the projection is on to the person of the analyst. A "positive" transference is the projection of images carrying constructive libido, a "negative" that of images carrying destructive libido. (Destructive libido may, however, be turned into "constructive" libido by a process of assimilation; that is, the constructive or destructive character of the psychic energy is determined by its function in the psychic process.) Projection is one of the most common psychic phenomena, both in analysis and outside it. As has been pointed out above, it is through projection that man becomes aware of inner processes which he does not notice otherwise. Thus it is of the greatest importance to realize in what way a projection on to another person or situation conceals one's own psychic activity. Withdrawal of projections is an act of self-recognition and is equivalent to becoming "conscious." Archetypal images are particularly apt to be projected. As long, for instance, as a boy projects the idea of "authority" completely on to the people around him—be it father or teacher—he is not yet aware of the archetype of the father, which among other contents also contains that of authority. The archetype represents the *inner* authority, the *inner* need for accepting and obeying an *immanent* law, instead of being subdued by external power. Similarly, as long as a man projects his "shadow"—i.e. his own primitive and negative side—on to some outside person or group of persons or circumstances, he is unaware of his own shadow figure. If he withdraws his shadow projections, he is face to face with his inner problem, and it is only then that the destructive energy of the projection can be transmuted into positive energy.

Exactly the same process takes place in analysis where the unconscious psychic contents are "transferred," i.e. projected on to the person of the analyst or the situation of analysis. For this reason, it is most important for the psychotherapist not to be drawn into a projection. If a patient dreams of some saviour, some man with supernatural powers and wisdom, and tries to explain to the analyst that he is this saviour, it would be utterly wrong for the analyst to accept this projection of the patient's inner image, i.e. of his archetype of the wise old man. He is to understand right from the beginning that this saviour is not the person of the analyst but his own inner potentiality. This means a refusal on the part of the analyst to accept a wrong suggestive power over the patient—which in any case would only be temporary.[1] But quite apart from the fact that it is only honest—and therefore in the long run much more constructive—not to accept what does not belong to one, it at least saves the analyst the embarrassment of having at another stage of the analysis to carry the burden of the projection of a destructive devil. The patient will be much more willing—and much better prepared—to accept his devil projection as an expression of his inner destructiveness if he has been handed back his saviour projection as his own precious possession. In this sense Analytical Psychology tends to discourage rather than encourage the transference situation. The realization of the analyst's human limitations and of his reality, and the consequent loss of "power," is in the last resort the patient's gain, and that is all that really matters.

* * *

Having laid down the main principles, I shall proceed to give a description of the approximate course of the analytical work; but I should emphasize once more that this is no more than an attempt to describe certain average conditions and methods of procedure which must and should be adapted and modified to suit every individual case.

The general introduction to an analysis consists in what is known as "anamnestic analysis," that is, a comprehensive anamnesis is made, filling in by careful questioning any gaps in the material which the patient himself provides. These gaps, considered from the analytical standpoint, are as a rule very characteristic, and with their help one can, by a little skilful questioning, bring within the patient's field of vision certain unapprehended

[1] It must, however, be pointed out that a situation might arise in which the patient *needs* his projection on to the analyst in order to be able to bear the burden of analysis; he cannot yet bear the reduction of the transference, and the analyst has therefore to accept the projection at least for some time. This point shows again how every "technique" can only describe the average procedure which may have to be modified according to the needs of a particular situation.

connections and associations if he is considered capable at this stage of facing them. The discussion of a patient's symptoms quite often provides the analyst at this stage of analysis with the most suitable opportunity of elucidating certain more superficial links. In other words, anamnestic analysis represents the reconstruction of the patient's biography and the development of his neurosis. In exceptional cases and with uncomplicated people, whose capacity and willingness to understand their inner motives is sometimes quite adequate, it may be possible by means of a few significant pointers directed at the psychic background of their disorder to pave the way at this early stage to a decisive alteration in their inner attitude.

Jung for instance quotes the following case:

"While acting as an officer in the Swiss Army Medical Corps, I often had occasion to apply this kind (the anamnestic analysis) of analytical method. For instance, a recruit, nineteen years old, reported sick with pains in the back. When I saw the young man he told me at once that he suffered from inflammation of the kidneys, and that the pain came from that malady. I asked him how he was able to diagnose his illness so definitely, whereupon he said that an uncle of his had the same trouble, and the same pains in the back. But further examination revealed no sign of any organic disease whatever. It was obviously a neurosis. I went into a careful investigation of the boy's recollections. The most important facts were that he had lost both his parents at a rather early age and that he lived with the uncle he had just mentioned. The uncle was his dearly-loved foster-father. The day before he reported sick, he had received a letter from the uncle, telling him that he was laid up again on account of his Bright's Disease. The letter affected him unpleasantly and he had thrown it away at once, without realizing the true character of the emotion he was thus trying to suppress. This emotion was really anxiety, a great fear that his foster-father might die, recalling his grief at the loss of his parents. When this unknown dread had been brought to the surface, the boy relieved his feelings by crying, with the result that the next morning he joined the ranks again. Here was an

identification with the uncle, made manifest by careful anamnesis. The realization of the suppressed emotion had a therapeutic effect."[1]

The anamnestic analysis is also very helpful in the treatment
of neurotic children, for whom dream analysis, on account of its
deep probing into the unconscious, is often not to be recommended. On the other hand, it will be obvious that in all the
more severe neuroses of adults (and also of children) anamnestic
analysis cannot represent the actual treatment, but is only an introduction to the true analysis of the unconscious. Anamnestic
analysis is only concerned with matters of which the patient is
either already conscious or which lie on the threshold of his consciousness. The interpretation then represents only a kind of
rearrangement of this material, and a better way of relating it to
conscious direction and control. The true analysis of the unconscious begins when the conscious contents have been exhausted.
This may happen very soon in the case of severe neuroses where
the patient puts up strong resistances to the probings of the
analyst and other ways of approach have therefore to be tried. It
is obviously impossible to give any stereotyped sequence since
anamnestic analysis and the analysis of the unconscious are likely
to overlap. At least this much may be said: that the analysis of the
unconscious is only possible when the conscious situation, as far
as it matters for the actual case, has been explored as far as possible. As the unconscious compensates the conscious side, an adequate picture of the latter has to be established before the unconscious material can be properly understood. The two main
functions of anamnestic analysis are thus to gain this picture of
the conscious situation, and to establish personal contact between patient and analyst, a contact which is of decisive importance. It also helps the patient to see his neurosis from a new
angle. Previously, his attention was directed wholly towards his
symptoms; it is now re-focused on the unconscious background
and history of the symptoms.

The relationship which has been established must not be con-

[1]Jung, *Contributions to Analytical Psychology*, p. 351f.

fused with transference in the technical sense, for it has nothing of its artificial and somewhat pathological character. It is rather the normal human rapport which is always necessary before two human beings can readily communicate with each other. Interference in a human being's unconscious constitutes such a hazardous and dangerous onslaught on his personality that the psychotherapist can only dare to do it if the contact between him and his patient is firmly rooted. For this reason, and because a dream reveals its meaning only against the background of the conscious situation, it is a grave mistake to start treatment by the analysis of a dream. Moreover, we must not overlook the fact that the way of treatment which Analytical Psychology has derived from its knowledge of the unconscious processes is to most people completely new and unfamiliar. So the patient needs, so to speak, a certain training before we can touch his unconscious material. Unconscious problems which may be capable of assimilation later on in the analysis, when the patient's relation to the analyst has become an Ariadne's thread which will bring him safely through the labyrinth, might at first cause him to react too violently and to protest by the simplest means at his command, namely by staying away.

A typical case in point is that of a clergyman who came to me because he felt that he had not used his creative powers to the best advantage. He felt dissatisfied with his general attitude to and progress in life. The discussion of his conscious situation had shown that he was a man full of ideals and theories which had, however, kept him much too much out of practical life and away from the acceptance of his concrete problems. Among those his marriage problem took an important place. He had tried all the time to deny the urgency of his concrete problems. His first dream, however, was this: "I was standing in a lavatory, my trousers in a heap on the floor at my side. A lady was coming towards me. I reflected that it was awkward. I was wearing no trousers, but fortunately I had on my pulpit gown." From his associations the sexual implication of this dream was clear, and so was the fact that he was using his pulpit gown, that is his "persona"—his social adaptation—to hide his problem and protect himself from its full impact. It was just this rejection of his instinctual problem which had prevented him from finding a satisfactory answer to life. That is why the dream apparently represented the compensatory side to his too high and abstract ideals. The atmosphere of the dream shows how the repressed instinct had taken on a regressive and negative character, and that until he faced up to this immediate and concrete problem, no satisfactory spiritual development could take place. When I pointed this out to him, he did not like it at all. He felt that he had not come to me for help over a sexual conflict, but on account of what he felt to be a certain sense of futility in his life. Although it was clear enough from the dream that the futility was closely connected with his sexual, and in a wider sense his instinctual problem, the true statement of facts as the dream gave it was too much for him. He decided to break off the analysis after a short time, because he felt that instead of dealing with his spiritual problem, I meant to discuss his sexual and relational problems.

This instance shows how important both a knowledge of the conscious situation and a secure foundation of personal contact are for the edifice of an analysis. In this particular case, the conscious problem had not been accepted and the foundations of personal contact had apparently not been laid. As on the other hand the patient's unconscious insisted on producing his instinctual problem so directly and right at the beginning, his ability or inability to face it was apparently the touchstone of how far it was possible for him to go through with the analysis altogether. In any case, this example shows how difficult it sometimes is to tolerate the impact of the unconscious.

Sometimes the unconscious chooses most impressive means to show the resistance. I remember the case of a young man of twenty-eight, the son of a famous father, who came from a background of a long-established and highly valued tradition. He arrived exactly half-an-hour late for his first interview. What had happened was that on his way to me he had parked his car at the college at which he studied a special subject rather against the wishes of his family. To him who came from a family with long connections with a very different kind of work from the one he had chosen for himself, the college symbolized his breakaway from the family tradition. He had parked his car in a rather careless way, so that he could really have foreseen what happened later. When he came out to drive on to my consulting-room, he found that another big car had been parked in front of his small one. After spending some time trying in vain to find the owner of the other car, he had to leave his blocked car there and come by taxi. I pointed out to him that his individuality had apparently been blocked by his collective sense of tradition, as it was really his carelessness which had produced the obstruction by the other car. He had to find new ways and means to come to me, and in this process he had shared his time exactly between the past and the future. Surprisingly enough he accepted this interpretation fairly easily; it seemed to "click," and thus a dangerous phase of resistance had been clarified before we really started.

Because of the decisive importance of the personal contact between analyst and patient, due regard must immediately be paid to the least sign of resistance. Such resistances often assume the oddest and most ridiculous forms. Thus I remember the case of a young patient of mine, aged twenty-one, who took three hours to overcome her resistance to giving expression to one of her notions. It was a hard fight between us, but in the end she admitted that what she couldn't stand about me was a certain old suit I sometimes wore. It sounds ridiculous, but such a battle nevertheless represents a decisive test of the strength of the relationship existing between patient and analyst. Any analyst who disregards the smallest resistance on the part of his patient or who treats it lightly, will unfailingly discover that the snowball will grow into an avalanche.

Once the anamnestic analysis, in addition to reproducing the history of the neurosis and acquainting the analyst with the present situation of the patient, has established a sure basis for the relationship between analyst and patient, the next step is to get into direct contact with the unconscious processes. For this the main line of approach is through the patient's dreams. The attitude of Analytical Psychology to dreams is very different from that of psychoanalysis. Freud himself once said: ". . . the dream is a pathological product, the first member of the series which includes the hysterical symptom, the obsession and the delusion among its members."[1]

Analytical Psychology, on the other hand, regards dreams as "the spontaneous self-portrayal in symbolical form of the actual state of the unconscious,"[2] and thus a dream gives a description of "the inner situation of the dreamer, the truth and reality of which the conscious mind will either not admit at all or only very unwillingly."[3] In other words, Freud looks on a dream as a pathological product from which the patient's complexes may be discovered, but which does not otherwise possess a meaning of its own. Jung, on the other hand, considers dreams an entirely natural and *normal* psychic function which can consequently act as a strongly positive and compensating force of considerable potential value. Thus the dream is not the symptom of pathological complexes but rather an attempt of the psyche to free the dreamer of his complexes. Analytical Psychology considers dreams not merely as a more or less sterile wish fulfilment or "complex-progeny," but as representing hitherto unacknowledged possibilities, previously neglected owing to a too onesided development of the personality. Nothing could show more clearly the profound difference between the attitude of psychoanalysis and that of Analytical Psychology than their respective points of view on the significance of dreams.

This difference in the point of departure of the two systems of analysis brings about a decisive difference in the practical handling of dream interpretation and in the whole method of exploring the unconscious. In the main there are two ways of approach:

[1]Freud, *New Introductory Lectures on Psychoanalysis.* Hogarth Press, London, 1937, p. 26.
[2]Jung, Allgemeine Gesichtspunkte zur Psychologie des Traumes, in: *Energetik der Seele,* Rascher, Zürich, 1928, p. 157.
[3]Jung, Die praktische Verwendbarkeit der Traumanalyse, in: *Wirklichkeit der Seele,* Rascher, Zürich, 1934, p. 73.

the analytical (or causal-reductive) interpretation ("analytical" being here used in the narrow sense of the word) and the synthetic or constructive interpretation. The causal aspect of the analytical interpretation tries to explain a symptom by reference to some definite experience or trauma in the past. It is mainly concerned with the history of a symptom, and consequently ascribes special value to the experiences of childhood, and to bringing them back into consciousness by the help of free associations. The reductive aspect of the analytical interpretation is not so much concerned with the biographical side of a symptom but, as its name says, with the reduction into its elements. This reduction is not necessarily causal and historical; its main purpose is to dispose of morbid and unsuitable "superstructures" in the conscious mind of the patient. This reduction may have to deal with very actual problems, or even with airy castles built into the future. The essential feature of such unsuitable superstructures is that they are built up to hide ulterior neurotic motives behind all kinds of illusions or perfectionist ideas; in other words that they are mechanisms of escape which have to be "debunked," before the psychic energy can be used in a truly constructive way.[1] (A case in question was that of the clergyman mentioned on page 35.)

It is obvious that in many cases we cannot dispense with the analytical method, both in its causal and its reductive aspects. It is especially necessary where a neurosis has been mainly caused by a conflict of the primary instincts; that is, it has to be used in cases where, and for as long as, the patient remains entangled in a web of conflicts which can be referred to infantile desires, whether they be sexual or power drives or whatever else, and where he tries to escape his real problems by illusory and futile "solutions." The main value of the analytical (causal-reductive) method lies therefore in three things; (1) that the attention of the patient is directed towards the unconscious psychological history of his illness; (2) that the patient is able to discover external facts which explain his subsequent illness; this helps him to lose his

[1]Cf. Jung, *Contributions to Analytical Psychology*, p. 360.

feelings of insufficiency and guilt, and thus calms and relieves the over-burdened psyche; and (3) that psychic energy which had been invested in the neurotic symptom in an inferior and destructive way is freed for future constructive use.

But this is only the first step; the further the analysis progresses, the more the attention should be diverted from external events experienced in childhood to the inner facts, that is, the fundamental and typical attitude towards life,[1] and the more the question arises what expression the newly gained energy is going to find. The movement inwards is of absolutely decisive importance for any true cure. In other words: when all is said and done, the important element in a neurotic conflict does not lie in the past but in the present, and the question which should therefore be asked is what essential task in life is the patient trying to evade. Here he may also find the constructive application for his "unfrozen" energies. Let us assume that a patient consults us because of a nervous breakdown. One can if one likes retrace the neurotic symptoms, for instance insomnia or an anxiety state, back into the past and pursue them right into infancy. That is, one can try to discover the causative factors, and in doing so one may elicit certain important disclosures, such as, for instance, that the patient had as a child certain alarming experiences which he is reliving in the present. But what one will not discover is why, and as we should say "what for," these possible traumata are breaking through again just now. This can only be done if, taking into consideration the actual present situation of the patient, one looks to the future and asks oneself: "What effect has this symptom? What does it either prevent or cause to happen?" One may then discover that the symptom is an attempt to force the patient into adopting a new attitude to life. For instance, Jung quotes the following case: "A man on the point of marrying an idolized woman of doubtful character, whose value he extravagantly overestimates, is seized with a spasm of the œsophagus, which forces him to a regimen of two cups of milk in the day, demanding his three-hourly attention. All visits to his fiancée are thus effectually

[1] Cf. the essay "Consciousness and Cure" in this volume.

stopped, and no choice is left to him but to busy himself with his bodily nourishment."[1] The symptom is in this interpretation not reduced to its first causes, it is not treated "historically" but understood from the point of view of its finality and prospective value.

In the interpretation of dreams the synthetic (constructive) method needs an approach that is fundamentally different from that of the analytical (causal-reductive) one. On the one hand the content of the dream can be reduced to "complexes of reminiscence" relating to objective or concrete situations or persons which are situated outside the dreamer. Jung has called this interpretation the interpretation on the objective level.[2] On the other hand, the images of the dream can be considered not as something concrete and outside the dreamer, but rather as "reflections of internal psychic factors and of the internal psychic situation of the dreamer";[3] this is interpretation on the subjective level.

This distinction is, strictly speaking, the same as that which was mentioned earlier[4] when the nature of projection was discussed. It is fundamentally the same thing as the difference between the situation of the child when he experiences authority—i.e. the power which controls his instinctual urges—as something that is imposed from outside, by the father, and when he has learned to see it as a function and a need of his own psyche. In each case the difference is whether contents of the psyche, such as the "shadow" or the "wise old man" are projected on to other people or whether they are realized as inner figures.

A short dream may illustrate the fundamental difference between the two interpretations. A man of forty-five dreams that he is riding in a car with a woman at the wheel. The woman leaves the car, and it immediately starts to run backwards and is very nearly wrecked by running into a wall. The dreamer feels in

---

[1] Jung: *Psychological Types*, p. 420f.
[2] Jung: *Two Essays on Analytical Psychology*, p. 87.
[3] Toni Wolff: *Einführung in die Grundlagen der Komplexen Psychologie*, p. 81; in *Die kulturelle Bedeutung der Komplexen Psychologie*, Springer, Berlin, 1935.
[4] Cf. pp. 30–32.

great danger without knowing how to deal with the situation, when the woman reappears and stops the car. A merely analytical interpretation would have to point out that the dreamer is apparently too dependent on the initiative of another person —presumably the mother—and that he has to take the wheel himself. This analytical interpretation would take the woman as a person outside the dreamer and is therefore an interpretation on the objective level. It would be justified, and indeed necessary, as long as the dreamer is too dependent upon external influences and leans too much on other people. This is normally the case in a younger person. The situation is, however, fundamentally different where independence of other people has been achieved. In that case the analytical-reductive interpretation on the objective level would miss the decisive point of the dream. As a matter of fact, this man was thoroughly adapted to external reality, as a man of forty-five should be. He had, however, reached a point where he had to face up to the as yet unsolved problem of the inner meaning of his life and of life in general. The message of the dream to him was that without the direction and help of the *inner* woman—the anima—his existence was menaced. He had to learn to accept the decisive importance and meaning of his unconscious (symbolized by the anima-figure) for the necessary re-orientation of his life. It is a re-orientation of quite a different nature from that which would be hinted at were the dream to be understood on the objective level. Not the adaptation to external, concrete reality —with which the analytical-reductive interpretation deals— was the problem of this man, but his adaptation to an inner psychic reality.

This example shows how the actual situation of the dreamer —and not some preconceived idea about the nature of his conflict, whether it be "nothing but" a problem of infantile sexuality, or of infantile power-drives—must always be the clue to the meaning of a dream. Accordingly both modes of interpretation, the analytical and the synthetic, have to be considered in each case, and that one has to be accepted which does most justice to the psychological position. It is not in the hands of the analyst to apply the one or the other interpretation in what might be in that case an arbitrary way, but it is the material that decides. Sometimes the situation may be quite ambivalent, and then all the analyst can do is to point out the two possibilities and watch the reaction, both conscious and unconscious. The analyst thus does not "make" the one or other interpretation; it is the material that is either reductive or prospective, or both. Both analyst and patient have to look round for the interpretation that "clicks." Then it will be seen which aspect of the interpretation creates an echo in the patient. With some patients one will find that the merely analytical interpretation does not or does not any longer produce any effect. On the other hand there are patients with whom a reductive interpretation works well enough. This interpretation alone will, it is true, not produce a full psychological integration and individuation, but for one thing some people may not be able to achieve this, and for another the main point of therapy is that the patient should be helped.

In any case the two interpretations are not mutually exclusive or contradictory but rather complementary. There is a common focal point in which both meet. This point is that as long as I am still tied to my personal father or mother, the realization and integration of the archetypal images of father and mother cannot take place. As long as the dreamer in the above-mentioned dream still suffers from a "mother fixation" he cannot achieve a creative relationship to his own unconscious, symbolized in the figure of the anima. Every problem which belongs to the layer of the personal unconscious blocks the corresponding experience of the image of the collective unconscious. Thus analytical-reductive and synthetic-constructive interpretation represent different stages of interpretation according to different stages of development. The analytical-reductive interpretation always proceeds on the objective level, whereas the synthetic-constructive one is an interpretation on the subjective level. The former has to reduce psychological facts to their elements, whether they be infantile instinctual drives, fixations, or other pathological complexes. It is necessary as long as personal problems stand between the dreamer and the super-personal, collective foundations of life. The synthetic interpretation, on the other hand, has to be applied in all cases "where either the conscious attitude is more or less normal but capable of greater development and differentiation, or where unconscious tendencies which are capable of development have been misunderstood or suppressed by the conscious mind."[1] It deals with irreducible and primordial psychic images existing in their own right, i.e. with archetypes.

It is obvious that with the constructive-synthetic approach the value of childhood recollections must become relative and limited. In the view of Analytical Psychology, their importance has been greatly exaggerated. Both analyst and patient spend laborious hours painstakingly angling in the dark waters of childhood recollections; they are very proud when they have hooked a particularly large or handsome fish, and nevertheless at the end of it all, things may be no better than they were. The mistake is that what is prior in time is regarded as also prior in value. From the point of view of Analytical Psychology, however, the present situation is regarded as more important both because of its irreducible immediate significance and because of its significance for the future.

*　　*　　*

Closely related to the different valuation of childhood recollections is a different attitude to the value of free associations. All that free associations can do is to reduce the dream elements to their underlying pathological complexes; they do not help to discover the meaning of the dream as such. It goes without saying that in elucidating a dream we also make use of the patient's associations, but usually from a different angle from that of psychoanalysis. To put it in a nutshell, it may be said that whereas psychoanalysis proceeds by means of free

[1] Jung, *Psychologie und Erziehung*, Rascher, Zürich, 1946, p. 76. Cf. also: *Contributions to Analytical Psychology*, p. 361.

association, Analytical Psychology works with a kind of controlled or "circular" association for the purpose of amplifying each element of a dream. This amplification results in an enrichment of the respective dream images by all possible analogous material through which the originally obscure dream becomes intelligible.[1] Instead of a chain of associations proceeding in a straight line and therefore capable of endless prolongation, this "controlled" association executes as it were a circling movement round the various components of a dream. In this way each link in the chain of associations is not merely determined by its predecessor, but also by its radial relation to the corresponding component of the dream itself. Thus one never loses sight of the original dream. In a diagram, the difference would appear as follows:

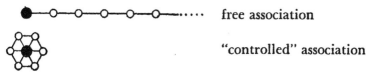

free association

"controlled" association

This kind of association is, as Jung has put it, like "a searchlight carefully and consciously directed on those associations which are grouped round the keyword of the dream." Supposing a dream contains the image of a tree or a door, we do not get our patient to go through an endless series of associations but ask him instead what this particular image "tree" or "door" *means* to him. Free association will doubtless enable one to put one's finger on the patient's complexes; but dreams are not necessary for this, because, as Freud rightly said, any casual thought may serve as the starting-point of associations which are rigidly determined by the subject's complexes. The circular method of association, on the other hand, utilizes any particular component of the dream not so much in order to discover complexes, but so as to find out what precise and individual meaning this component possesses in this particular

[1] Cf. Jung, *The Integration of the Personality*, Kegan Paul, London, 1940, p. 207. For an elaborate example of the method of amplification cf. the "Study of a Dream" in this volume.

dream context.[1] Free associations are needed if it is thought
necessary by means of them to find out the hidden latent
meaning of a dream behind the disguise of the manifest dream.
But since Analytical Psychology does not accept this theory
of the distortion of the meaning of a dream, it arrives at a
different valuation of free associations. To express it briefly:
while Freud asks "What is the dream caused by? What is it a
symptom of?" Jung asks "What is the meaning of the dream?
What is it a *symbol* of?"

This distinction expresses once more a deep-seated difference
in Jung's and Freud's conception of the nature of the unconscious. If, with Freud, one considers all dreams pathological,
one will confine one's interest to the disorder, that is the
pathological complexes, in these dreams; whereas if, with Jung,
one looks on dreams as the normal and creative self-expression
of the unconscious, one's interest is concentrated on the meaning
of the dream itself. The creative nature of the unconscious is
still apparent in a neurosis and its symptoms. As has been pointed
out before, they represent an attempt, although an unsuccessful one, to regulate the deranged balance of the psyche. The
task of analytical treatment—and of dream-interpretation as a
part of it—is therefore to help the patient to find out the positive
and progressive tendencies behind the unadapted and consequently unsuccessful attempt at compensation. All these points
may be illustrated by the following characteristic example.

A man, aged fifty-one, complains that for some time now,
whenever he travels by train or aeroplane and the speed goes
beyond a certain limit, he gets attacks of giddiness and falls a
victim to uncontrollable feelings of anxiety. One can, if one
chooses, lay all the emphasis on his early history; that is, one
can try to ascertain what actual trauma the patient sustained
in his childhood or what painful adolescent experience he is
repressing. On the other hand, one may proceed on quite different lines; namely by starting from the present acute situation
in which this symptom is making itself felt. In other words: one

[1]An example of this "controlled" association is given on p. 76f.

may use either the reductive or the synthetic approach. Let me present the case from the second angle. This man was a successful and happily married business man, just at the beginning of his fifties, and was himself quite unable to suggest any reason for his symptoms. The only thing he could suggest was that these absurd "hysterical" attacks, as he condescendingly called them, were particularly annoying since his business necessitated frequent and lengthy journeys. Thus he had recently been obliged to send one of his subordinates to an important conference because he himself was too frightened to undertake the train journey.

If one begins questioning him with a view to unearthing the causative agency in his past history, one may possibly discover that the patient suffered a shock as a child which was associated with giddiness; but that will certainly not tell one why this trauma is making itself felt again at this precise moment. Thus, in actual fact, one will be scarcely any better off than one was before. For it is precisely this present moment in time that matters. But if one takes a finalistic view and considers the present acute position from the point of view of its future possibilities, one will immediately perceive that the symptoms have one definite and immediate effect, since it is obvious that the patient's sensations of giddiness and the accompanying fear considerably curtail his business activities. Apart from the inherently unpleasant symptoms, it is precisely this diminution of his capacity for work which has caused the patient to consult a psychotherapist. Yet, if we take this apparent disability of his to represent an unsuccessful attempt at adaptation, the symptoms point to something quite other, namely to a strong secret desire to escape from his business engagements.

At this point it is necessary to guard against a possible misunderstanding. A similar explanation might be given by the school of Alfred Adler's Individual Psychology, namely that the symptom is an attempt to cut loose from his business duties; but Individual Psychology would interpret this in the negative sense as an attempt at escape. Analytical Psychology, on the other hand, taking into account the particular circumstances of the patient, as, for instance, his age, has to interpret it positively as a purposeful signpost pointing to an inner necessity in his life. That is, subject to correction or later reconsideration as the result of further talks with the patient, I should explain the symptoms as follows. This man has identified himself so completely with his business life and social duties that the balance of his psyche has been seriously disturbed. His symptoms are an unconscious attempt to force him to restrict to reasonable proportions his altogether excessive over-valuation of business and social life. As he is over fifty, i.e. definitely in the second half of life, his external activities should gradually be curtailed. From the practical standpoint alone, we should therefore not try to investigate his childhood recollections or traumata, but, basing ourselves on a very simple and direct explanation of his main symptoms, try to put our finger on the weak point in his present situation.

I should like to relate a later dream of the patient's, which illustrates the same symptom from another angle. "It is harvest time; I am sitting on a large wagon, laden with hay, which I am driving back to the barn, but the load of hay is so high that the lintel of the door into the barn knocks me on the head, so that I fall off my seat and I wake up terrified in the act of falling." The meaning of the dream approached from the prospective angle is clear; obviously the patient has overloaded his wagon to such an extent that he exceeds his capacity, and as a consequence his conscious intentions receive a blow. The task of the analysis consists, therefore, in making the dreamer aware of this message of his unconscious, and this awareness will help him to establish a right relation between outer success and inner need. In other words, this dream has to be understood as an attempt of his psyche to compensate for the one-sided extraverted attitude, which, having regard to his position in the second half of life, goes against the real psychological rhythm and therefore disturbs his balance. One of the central conceptions of Analytical

Psychology is clearly illustrated by this case: that of the psyche as a self-regulating system. Wherever the psychological situation of an individual has become unbalanced by a too extreme or one-sided attitude, wherever his essential needs have been disregarded or neglected, the unconscious tends to produce the material that is necessary to restore the balance and wholeness of that situation. In this sense, the unconscious has a constant influence on and relationship to the conscious mind. These may, however, be overlooked or depreciated by the exaggerated conscious position. It is then that "symptoms" occur, and the energetic function of these, rightly understood, is that of a danger signal. The unconscious psyche in its deep impersonal layers has, as it were, a judgment on the situation which is not distorted by fear, ambitions, desires, fixations or whatever the case may be; but is interested in restoring the balanced pattern of the individual. That is why Jung has called the unconscious the "objective psyche," as it plays a superior and detached rôle in regard to the possible distortions of the conscious mind with its subjective prejudices.

It is unnecessary to stress the difficulty which a number of patients experience in acknowledging the truth of this kind of interpretation of their breakdown. Instead of helping them to rout round among their childhood recollections for a scapegoat by means of which to rid themselves of their responsibility for their symptoms, the analyst confronts them with what in the last resort is an ethical claim to self-examination and a re-orientation of their personal life. But we can obviously not allow ourselves to be put off by any such resistances. It happens only too often that a patient expects at the begining of an analysis that the psychotherapist will, by some magical means, simply rid him of his symptoms without ever touching the rest of the structure of his life, with which he is quite satisfied. The analyst is only too often supposed to be a kind of "medicine man," who will make the symptom disappear from outside. The truth is that nobody can be cured unless he is prepared to accept the need for a more or less complete re-orientation of his life. To put it in a nutshell: the healed person is not the original person minus a symptom, but a newly orientated person in whom, through the new orientation, the necessity for the symptom, and therefore the symptom itself, has disappeared. It may even sometimes happen that a cure does not mean the disappearance of a symptom, but that instead it makes the suffering caused by the symptom disappear, because the original suffering has fulfilled its purpose.

It might be illuminating to examine the above dream of the hay wagon both from the Freudian and the Adlerian point of view, i.e. from an exclusively reductive and analytical angle. In the first case, the barn would have to be taken as a symbol for the female genitalia, and the dream would therefore be interpreted as a tendency towards regression into the maternal womb, a tendency which, because of its undercurrent of incestuous desire, would be followed by punishment (castration). The interesting and important point is that, at a certain level, this explanation is entirely justified, for the stifling of the unconscious possibilities of a human being arises often enough, especially in the case of a man, from an unresolved mother fixation. Such a fixation, in which the mother still exercises an unconscious spell, threatens to impede the normal development of the ego. One possible answer to this is to reject the mother completely and to over-emphasize the ego side, and with it the rational "conscious," and (in the sociological sense) collective values. Behind the personal mother, however, there is hidden the mother-archetype, which is the symbol of the unconscious, i.e. the non-ego. This non-ego, on account of the fear of (and the unconscious domination by) the personal mother, is felt to be hostile. In other words, the personal mother and the mother-archetype are still not separated from each other, and out of fear of the personal mother the deeper and constructive significance of the mother-archetype is missed. The over-emphasis on the ego-attitude and the rejection of the unconscious, however, are bound to lead to an impasse.

A merely reductive attitude deals only with the personal mother-fixation, and it needs the constructive and synthetic attitude to contact the creative potentialities in the unconscious, i.e. the images of the collective unconscious. The fixation to and the fear of the personal mother is then seen to have concealed the deeper problem of the relationship to the mother-archetype. This mother-archetype is the first form of the anima-experience, and what matters to the patient is the achievement of a positive relationship to the anima, i.e. to his unconscious. This shows how a merely reductive interpretation, unless completed by the constructive one, remains but an unsatisfactory torso.

If, on the other hand, the dream is examined from the standpoint of Individual Psychology, it will have to be interpreted as showing an exaggerated will to power, compensating for an inherent inferiority complex. This explanation too contains a certain element of truth, as every incompleteness of the personality such as is bound to result from an infantile fixation produces a feeling of inferiority; but it also is lacking in constructive and progressive values, the reason being that both the Freudian and the Adlerian explanation have left out of account the compensating and positive elements in the dream. This dream example is interesting because it shows how different explanations may be relatively true on different levels and from different angles. But the whole point consists in finding the interpretation which goes home, includes most, and has most meaning to the patient, and thus offers most hope for reconstructive work in the future.

This method of dream interpretation occasionally enables, and indeed sometimes requires the analyst to enlarge upon the patient's associations by means of his own knowledge. This is especially the case when the dream contains archetypal images, the significance of which must of necessity be out of reach of the dreamer's conscious knowledge.[1] But it goes without saying that our contribution is legitimate and useful only when the dreamer is in complete agreement with it. In fact, it may be stated generally that the interpretation of a dream is valid only when the dreamer can accept it fully, that is when it "means" something to him. Moreover, the only way to avoid conscious suggestions is

[1] Cf. the essay "Study of a Dream" in this volume.

that we should consider any interpretation of a dream invalid and insufficient until we can find a formula to which the dreamer himself can give his entire assent. It need hardly be said that this does not mean allowing the patient to get away with resistances and subterfuges. Yet there is a very real difference between an attempt to shirk the issue of a dream and an honest inability to accept an interpretation, even if it should be thoroughly justified and correct from the analyst's point of view, or rather from the point of view of his theory.

Thus it can happen—and does happen quite frequently—that the analyst gives an interpretation which is "correct," or is proved at a later stage of the analysis to have been correct, and nevertheless it has to be admitted that at that earlier stage the interpretation was *psychologically* wrong. The practical importance of a dream is that through the fact of its being understood and integrated, some of the energy of the unconscious becomes attached to the conscious mind, and that thus the potential of consciousness is raised. For this reason Jung has called the symbol a transformer of energy: the unconscious energy which is unassimilable in the form of neurotic symptoms is transformed into energy which can be integrated into the conscious attitude by means of a symbol, whether it be of a dream or any other form in which the unconscious expresses itself. It is therefore the ego which has to assimilate the energy brought within the range of consciousness by a dream, and unless the ego is prepared for this process of integration, it cannot take place.

Thus, for instance, dreams of psychotics and sometimes of children, although they are full of constructive potentialities, cannot fulfil their rôle, because the integrative power of the ego is insufficient or the gap between the ego and the unconscious too great. One of my patients, a schizophrenic, produced dream after dream in which he *almost* achieved an integrative step, but something was always lacking. Two typical dreams were these: "I found myself in the company of others, in the crater of a vast extinct volcano, containing many other similar extinct volcanoes and one that was still active. The scenery round me was grey and desolate, and nothing living could possibly exist there for any length of time. I walked to the edge of the crater, and on looking over saw a street that resembled Regent Street. Some of the others with me had suitcases and were able to descend easily. After a time, I was able to shout, *but I was unable to descend into the street.*" And the other: "I was being attacked by a mob, and was in great danger of being destroyed by them. At the same time, I could see, coming to my rescue or walking towards me, though in another part of the town, a tall straight figure, dressed in white. . . . The mob carried me to a wall and pushed me up it. *The white figure did not arrive.*"

Both dreams show the agonizing nearness of rescue which nevertheless just does not "arrive." It *should* be possible to achieve integration, but in practice the gap between the danger and the rescue cannot be bridged. It is as if the unconscious images are quite detached from the dreamer's conscious personality; as though he is so foreign to himself that he is no longer a concern of himself. The gap between his unconscious and his conscious mind has become too wide, and thus the unconscious symbols can no longer be assimilated by his ego.

This extreme case underlines the need for keeping the particular situation of the dreamer firmly in mind. In the case of the neurotic, the integration *can* be achieved, but dreams may anticipate possible solutions which at present are beyond the reach of the dreamer. The interpretation of every dream has therefore to be adapted to the concrete situation and potentialities of the dreamer, and no interpretation, however correct theoretically, can disregard this fact. Thus the honest assent to or rejection of an interpretation by the dreamer—that is, his indication of how far he can at that stage assimilate his own unconscious— is the most valuable corrective for the psychotherapist.

It should again be emphasized that what is given here is merely a general plan of the usual procedure in Analytical Psychology, and that just as anamnestic analysis and the analysis of the unconscious can shade off into one another, so it is with the analytical-reductive and the synthetic-constructive interpretation of a dream, only more so. There may be occasions when it is imperative to make the constructive interpretation precede the reductive one, or it may happen in certain cases that even with the technique of Analytical Psychology, the reductive interpretation will occupy the greater part of the time. The position is rather like that in geology. A completely clear definition of geological strata may be possible in a certain landscape, and still, on account of dislocations and breakages of the strata, it will happen that if the geologist goes down into the earth, he will find that the different strata present themselves in a different and much more complex order. Clear definitions and logical categories are characteristics of the conscious mind, but not of the unconscious which is spontaneous and non-rational, like nature.

Just because Analytical Psychology endeavours to establish a synthesis between the analytical-reductive and the synthetic-constructive interpretations, which are in its view twin aspects of one whole, it is difficult to lay down any hard-and-fast rules for any given case. This is, however, not the only occasion in psychotherapy where general rules must be modified in practice according to each particular situation, and where in consequence the final "technique" has to be modified through the experience and intuition of the individual psychotherapist. For reasons which have been explained above, however, Analytical Psychology usually considers the analytical-reductive interpretation as being the more superficial one, and the synthetic-constructive interpretation as penetrating much more deeply into the heart of the problem; though the two are complementary to one another and not mutually exclusive. The danger inherent in a purely analytical-reductive conception consists in its neglect of the progressive tendencies in the unconscious, as they are forced into the light of day by the very conflict itself; a neglect which produces a devaluation and destruction of vital values. On the other hand, the danger of concentrating all one's attention on the constructive issues is that by so doing one may neglect the elementary conflict of instincts and stimulate the patient to produce a crop of phantasies which he finds himself unable to translate into reality. In the last resort, a right judgment on the use of these methods can only be obtained if the analyst himself has experienced their dynamics on himself. This makes it absolutely imperative for an analyst to be analysed himself (as does, of course, the necessity that the analyst himself should be, as far as is humanly possible, "conscious" and integrated, that is, aware of his own problems and proof against the danger of projecting them on to a patient).

It has been stated above that, generally speaking, the analytical-reductive interpretation comes first, and the synthetic-constructive one at a later stage. In this connection, something must be said about the analyst's general attitude to the patient at the beginning and during the course of the analysis. It goes without saying that as the analysis proceeds and above all towards its end, an endeavour is made to loosen the patient's dependence on the analyst. This is done mainly by laying increasing emphasis on independent action by the patient. In theory this means that whereas at the beginning the analyst assumes complete responsibility and acts, so to speak, as the patient's externalized consciousness—i.e. he has to carry the projection of the patient's mature personality—in the later stages the patient is led once more to assume this discriminating function himself. In practice this means that increasing emphasis is laid on the patient learning to analyse himself and to handle his own unconscious material. This is done partly by using the technique of active imagination, which will be explained more fully later, and partly by getting the patient to work out his associations to his dreams carefully before he comes to the interview. He thus brings the analyst the dream and its context, so that all that remains to be done is for the analyst and patient together to clarify and interpret the results. At a still later stage, it may even be considered desirable for the patient himself to learn to analyse at least the simpler and more transparent of his dreams, as well as his symptomatic actions.

Another way to increase the patient's self-reliance and independence is to lengthen the intervals between the interviews towards the end of the analysis, reducing their number from say three to two, and later one a week. Eventually still longer intervals in the treatment may be introduced. Moreover, the introduction of such intervals before the final termination of the analysis provides the patient with a kind of bridge so that in the event of an occasional relapse his confidence in the treatment remains unshaken. It is best to discharge the patient on probation, so to speak, and to arrange for him to come to report from time to time. In actual practice, this may mean fairly prolonged after-treatment, but only at long intervals which can be adjusted to individual needs. The value of educating the patient so that he is capable of a certain amount of self-analysis becomes practically apparent at this stage.

*   *   *

An important part of analysis, particularly in its later stages, is the technique of active imagination. This "technique" plays a very characteristic and specific part in the method of Analytical Psychology, and it will therefore be considered in some detail, in spite of the great difficulty of attempting to describe it at all adequately in a short space and to somebody who has not experienced it himself. Strictly speaking, the word "technique" is wrong in connection with these processes of active imagination, just as one can hardly speak of a "technique of dreaming." Dreams are natural events, and so are the images of active imagination. If the word "technique" is used in this connection, it has therefore to be understood only as referring to the technique of *perceiving* these images, just as we may give people some technical advice on how to remember or observe their dreams, i.e. by showing them or helping them to find out what is the best attitude in the face of such psychic facts.

By "active imagination" we understand a definite attitude towards the contents of the unconscious, whereby we seek to isolate them and thus observe their autonomous development. We may also say that we "make them come to life," but this is incorrect in as far as we merely observe what is happening. The right attitude may perhaps be best described as one of "active passivity." That is, one keeps completely passive and receptive to what is going to emerge from one's own unconscious, but at the same time focuses one's attention actively on what is going to happen. It is not unlike watching a film or listening to music, where in each case one sits back and "takes in" something which one has not made but which happens, with a concentration which is a definite kind of activity. Only the difference is that in active imagination the "film" is being unrolled inside.

Let us take for example a dream in which the dreamer undergoes a certain alarming experience, such as, for instance, shipwreck, after which he finds himself swimming about absolutely alone in a dark ocean. Or we can take a phantasy image where the patient feels that he is being threatened by a shrouded figure enveloped in dark veils. One may suggest to the patient that he should concentrate on one or other of these situations. In the case of most people, with the expenditure of a little time and practice, these situations, or, as we might more aptly term them, these mental images, show a certain autonomous life and movement; they develop and acquire added characters. In short, if we concentrate on them, they form the nucleus for a group of other contents of the unconscious which gather round them. For instance, in the first example of a shipwreck, the sudden appearance of an island may spell safety, or, on the other hand, the situation may become even worse owing to yet another danger cropping up. In the second example, the menacing figure may acquire recognizable features. These new details furnish most valuable information about the background and the meaning of the original image.

It will be easier to understand what is happening in such a situation if we keep in mind that a neurosis can be defined as "a dissociation of personality due to the existence of complexes."[1] A complex is a constellation of psychic contents charged

[1] Jung, "Fundamental Psychological Conceptions," a Report on five lectures, given under the auspices of The Institute of Medical Psychology, printed as MS. London, 1936, p. 212.

with emotional energy. It is important to remember that the psychic contents are not always identical with repressed or unconscious contents. For one thing, one can talk of the centre of the conscious mind, the ego, as a psychic complex, in as far as it represents a definite constellation of emotional energy round a certain nucleus, which acts as a centre of gravity. For another thing, there are complexes which, although they are unconscious, are not repressed but merely not yet conscious; that is, they represent future potentialities of the personality which have not yet reached the threshold of consciousness.

Thus "to have complexes" does not necessarily mean to be pathological. Everyone has complexes, for to have a complex means no more than to possess certain dynamic and emotionally charged psychic centres of gravity, which because of their emotional force attract and act as foci for other psychic experiences. We only begin to speak of a neurosis when certain of these emotionally charged psychic factors or complexes are not, or do not appear to be, compatible with the general trend of the personality, and consequently cause a more or less deep split or dissociation. The essential feature of every complex is that it absorbs psychic energy. If a complex is located in the unconscious, it attracts energy which should be at the disposal of the conscious personality. Thus it causes a minus in adaptation and consequently a neurotic disturbance appears, whether the symptom be psychological or physical. The task of analysis consists in bridging the dissociation, that is in an integration or re-integration of the different parts of the personality.

If the complex is not a repressed but rather an as yet subliminal content, it will be found to conceal the progressive potentiality of the personality behind its neurotic manifestation. This means, as has been pointed out before, that a neurosis is a so far unsuccessful attempt at a re-orientation of the personality. Therefore it is always of paramount importance, and indeed absolutely necessary, to seek the positive meaning behind a symptom or complex. A complex is like a fragmentary personality of its own, and not only must it be taken as such, but the patient

COMPARATIVE STUDY OF ANALYTICAL PSYCHOLOGY

also must be taught to look at and to relate to it in this light. The idea that a complex is something like a separate personality may seem strange, but it will become clearer from the example which follows. Active imagination is a means of getting into touch with these "personalities" and of integrating their hidden progressive energies. A small episode which contains in a nutshell the whole meaning of the complex and its reintegration by active imagination may help to illustrate this. It is the case of a young girl of twenty-three, who was suffering from insomnia. She was so completely under the domination of her mother that she might, with justice, be said to be psychologically still unborn. Of course she was quite unaware of this, and so was her mother. At an early stage of the treatment I asked my patient, whom we will call Joan, if she could suggest any possible reason for her insomnia. After a good deal of opposition, she finally admitted that she was afraid of going to sleep because when she closed her eyes, a grey figure used to appear beside her bed. It was one of those typical cases of insomnia which are due to the fear of surrendering to a state of unconsciousness, because the patient is afraid of the unconscious images which may emerge once conscious control is relaxed. Thus he prefers a state of relative sleeplessness to the "dangerous" loss of control in sleep. At that stage my patient had learned one thing at any rate: that she was afraid to go to sleep. This, together with the fact that she was an essentially unneurotic type, induced me to risk a frontal attack. I asked her to describe this grey figure to me as minutely as possible. I did *not* ask her for free associations which might have led away from the figure rather than revealed its true nature. Her resistance to my request was so decided that at first hardly any advance could be made on these lines. We did, however, get at least as far as to establish that the figure was that of a woman, and that her face was entirely concealed. In order to get beyond this point, I asked my patient the name of the woman. This question came as a complete surprise, and seemed quite stupid to her. She told me that *of course* she did not know the name, and how could she possibly, etc. I held on, however, and reminded her that some people play at giving names to people who are walking down the street in front of them, and I suggested that she should try to do the same with her grey woman, whereupon she suddenly fell into a terrific rage and without a moment's hesitation burst out "Damn it all, her name is Joan." One has to remember—that was her own name. The result was astonishing; after her sudden access of "anger," which was in reality a sudden influx of libido out of the unconscious complex into the conscious mind—she broke into a long fit of weeping. The surprise attack had broken down the barrier between her unconscious complex and her conscious mind. All of a sudden, the patient had realized that she was confronted with her own dormant individuality, which claimed recognition, and consequently demanded a re-orientation and readjustment of her life. This individuality had been hidden underneath her identification with her mother. She had been afraid of the responsibilities of her own independent and adult life, and thus had so far successfully managed to overlook the claim of her individuality. Her insomnia was gone from this moment, although the achieving of independence from her mother took a good deal of time.

This perhaps rather unimpressive example contains all the elements of active imagination. More than that, it shows the specific difference between the approach of Analytical Psychology and that of other psychotherapeutic methods. The root conception which gives the approach of Analytical Psychology its specific character, and which indeed forms the foundation on which its whole technique is built, is the absolute directness and seriousness with which it accepts the reality of the unconscious and its contents as an essential part of the whole personality. For it the unconscious is, as Jung has so often pointed out, not merely "nothing but," that is, nothing but repressed sexuality or repressed will to power; but, as the matrix of the conscious mind, it is the really potent and creative layer of our psyche. The unconscious contains all the factors which are necessary for the integration of the personality. It possesses, as it were, a superior knowledge of our real needs in regard to their integration and the ways to achieve them.

Only when the unconscious is understood in this way as the "objective psyche," containing all the regulating and compensating factors which work for the wholeness of the personality, does it make sense to advise a patient to face his unconscious in such a direct and forceful manner. A similar "technique" can be used by those who hold quite different views, but in that case it will be a technique only and not the living expression of a synthetic and constructive psychology, as opposed to a merely analytical and reductive one. For instance, the effect produced in the case of insomnia, mentioned above, was not due to the fact that the figure which the patient saw was suddenly endowed with her name—on the contrary, this alone might have plunged the patient even more deeply into her neurosis. Her release was due to the fact that, by naming it as she did, she realized in a flash the right of this still completely shrouded phantom—the symbol of her adult personality—to recognition and to a life of its own.

Moreover, her action in giving it a name also established contact between her conscious mind and her "autonomous complex." For to name a thing is more than a superficiality: the name is the symbol for the essence and substance of a thing or a person, and therefore possesses a "magic" quality. This is well known from countless fairy tales and legends, and Oscar Wilde makes one of his characters say: "When I like people immensely, I never tell their names to anyone. It is like surrendering a part of them." Her own "complex" had thus revealed its true nature to her, and instead of an attitude of fear and panic—which had caused her insomnia—one of acceptance and relatedness could be created.

Considered carefully, this episode thus contains the germ of all that we understand by the term "active imagination." The next step, which for certain reasons I did not take in this case, might have been to advise my patient to start a regular conversation, in the form of question and answer, with this grey woman.

But this technique of conversation with the personified contents of one's unconscious presupposes a considerable psychological maturity. It needs a capacity for detachment and surrender at the same time, which is not easy to attain, let alone that in such a conversation things may come out which the one partner in the discussion, i.e. our ego, finds it difficult to digest, and which may indeed cause a dangerous shock. For all these reasons, it is often as well not to make use of this technique of conversation until fairly late in the analysis.

Of course, it is often difficult for us modern Western people who pride ourselves so tremendously on the supremacy of our conscious will, to accept these processes which we can see developing, or rather just taking place in the unconscious when we watch carefully, and not to believe that they are simply artificial products intentionally invented and created by our conscious selves. How difficult it is for most people to believe that dreams or slips of the tongue are not merely meaningless chance products but on the contrary are the expression of purposeful psychic processes.

One of the chief objections made against the results of active imagination is that we add deliberately, or rather by a process of self-deception, to the original image—in brief, that we *make* these further images or events appear and that they are not a spontaneous self-development of the original image itself. One answer to this objection is the convincing sense of self-evident reality which active imagination conveys to the person who experiences it. Another answer is provided by the fact that these processes of active imagination possess an autonomy which is most surprising. One finds very frequently that things happen contrary to everything which one expected, that one is overcome by a sudden panic in face of the development of the image, and yet one is forced to accept what happens by the weight and dynamic power of the inner process. Likewise one feels that one would like to see a certain thing, for instance a face, more clearly, and one simply cannot force the unconscious to reveal that face.

This gives an absolutely convincing feeling of these processes as being independent of the desires or fears or expectations of one's own ego. The decisive fact is that these inner images are not of our own making, but that they reveal an inner psychic life to us. Thus active imagination must be regarded as a process of contemplation of, or meditation on, unconscious images. All we *do* is to provide concentrated attention, and submission to and reverent observation of the inner images. To redirect the libido is all we do actively about it, just as we do in every concentrated and detached observation of facts.

When describing the method of using active imagination, I mentioned that if a person concentrates on the images thrown against the screen of the psychic background, these images begin to come to life. There are, however, other ways in which the technique of active imagination can be used, above all in drawing. Again and again one will find that patients when relating dreams exclaim: "I saw it all so clearly, I ought really to draw it." Obviously these people feel that mere words are quite inadequate to express the vivid experiences which they had lived through either in a dream or phantasy. They feel the need of giving expression to the inner experience by some different means of a symbolical nature. The inner experience has been so powerful and impressive, its content transcends words to such an extent, that another more adequate expression has to be found.

This can easily be understood if we think of the use of symbols, for instance in religion. The very existence of such symbols means that an experience has taken hold of people which eludes rational definition. A symbol is *not* a sign for something that can just as well be expressed in rational words. That is why Freud really uses the term "symbol" incorrectly. A stick, for instance, is not a symbol for a sex organ, but merely a sign or a cypher; his "symbol" does not in any way express more than can also be expressed in another and a rational way. A true symbol, however, as for instance the cross in Christianity, expresses considerably more than a rational and known fact. It is not, as with Freud, a static sign, but a dynamic experience. Where a symbol is needed as expression of an experience, every other mode of expression

would be inadequate. An archetypal content which breaks
through into the conscious psyche is still too powerful, too full
of irrational significance for the conscious mind to grasp its meaning fully, and therefore it cannot be adequately defined. The
energy of the symbol is thus derived precisely from the fact that
it expresses in an image an experience which on account of its
complexity and uniqueness eludes intellectual formulation. This
does not, of course, mean that the conscious mind cannot be affected by these contents in a constructive sense; it only means
that the conscious mind cannot formulate them sufficiently.
Once they are fully analysed and formulated, they lose their original significance as symbols. Symbols are a kind of numinous
energetic phenomenon, and exercise a strong influence on the
conscious psyche beyond the possibility of defining them. They
are expressions of archetypal events, prior to differentiation or
rationalization. As such, they help to lead over the energy of the
archetype into the conscious mind. For this reason, symbols have
the capacity of controlling undifferentiated and primitive libido.
They are "the invaluable means by which we are able to use for
effective work the merely instinctive flow of the energetic process."[1] This explains the great significance of symbols in every
religion, where they serve as expressions, channels and transformers of the experience of the highest numinous archetype of
the deity. Psychologically speaking, the immediate experience
of the archetype of the deity means such an enormous influx of
energy that the conscious personality is in danger of being ex-
ploded.[2] A symbol is therefore always the attempt to formulate
an archetypal experience as adequately as possible for the use
of the conscious mind (a definition which again shows the tremendous gap that separates psychoanalysis from Analytical Psychology). As Jung has said, "The mythological image, indefinite
and yet definite, and the iridescent symbol express the psychic
process more aptly, more fully, and therefore infinitely more
clearly than the clearest concept; for the symbol does not only

---

[1] Jung, *Contributions to Analytical Psychology*, p. 52.
[2] Cf. the essay "The Psychological Approach to Religion" in this volume.

give us a representation of the process, but also—and this is perhaps equally important—enables us to share in or to live in retrospect the experience of the process. Such a process is a twilight phenomenon which we can only understand by a sympathetic participation . . . but never by a heavy-handed interference which wants to make everything clear."[1]

If, therefore, a patient feels the urge to make a drawing—or any other similar representation of a dream or phantasy—he does so because the experience in the dream or phantasy on the one hand transcends his power of rational formulation, and, on the other, because he feels the need to connect this experience with his conscious mind as far as possible. This also explains why symbols, just as dreams do, change their meaning in the course of years, as they reveal ever-new facets to the conscious mind.

The symbolical presentation of the original unconscious experience may be more or less beyond the patient's understanding; and yet, by the very fact that it has been produced, it nevertheless exerts an integrating influence, because, as was explained above, a channel has been created for the gradual integration of the unconscious energy and content. Symbols thus created and shaped have a strong reflex action on the patient, since the meditation and contemplation directed towards them has an integrative effect in itself.

This effect is shown in the following case, which has several interesting features. For one thing, it illustrates again how autonomous these unconscious processes are and answers the objection that they are more or less arbitrary products of little value. Secondly, it shows how a symbolical theme is used to represent an inner development that has taken place during a period of analysis. Finally, it will show how the symbolical representation that grows out of the psychological process may far transcend the limitations and resources of the conscious mind.

The case in question is that of a young woman of twenty-eight who had come to me because of severe depressions and dissociations, together with suicidal tendencies. Treatment lasted for

[1] Jung, *Paracelsica*, Rascher, Zürich, 1942, p. 135.

about two years, and in addition to the intensive work which was
done on her dreams, her drawings became increasingly important. The patient produced about sixty of these drawings, of
which I propose to discuss four. The first two pictures are the
first the patient ever made, while the third one was produced
about two months later, and the fourth near the end of her analysis. The analysis had gone on for about five months, and a good
deal of personal history had been related which turned to a large
extent on her relationship to her father. He had apparently been
a most unpleasant person, and her relationship to him had been
correspondingly bad. Her mother had died when she was about
ten years old, and her father a year later. After her mother's death,
she had been brought up by a governess who was tyrannical and
pedantic, and my patient, who was a very sensitive and highly intuitive girl, had been affected severely by all these unfavourable
circumstances. Her individual development had been seriously
interfered with, and she suffered from strong feelings of inferiority and insufficiency. The first months of analysis were
largely a battle for a relationship with me—which she needed
badly as a counter-weight to her bad relationship with her
father in particular, and her mistrust of human relationships in
general—and a fight against a feeling of complete hopelessness
with regard to her own future and her own potentialities. Then
suddenly, after about five months, she brought, without any suggestion of mine, the first picture (cf. picture 1, page 32).

It represents a kind of cemetery with three graves, of which
the central one with its enormous tombstone is specially prominent. The atmosphere of the picture as a whole is very sinister
and murky, and in the air there are ghostly faces, pistols, poison
bottles and similar unpleasant objects. I want to deal only with
the most important problem of this picture, as expressed in the
central grave. On the tombstone are written a great number of
words: "Father—uncle—mother—guilt—child—witch—madness—profession—analysis—gas—man—death—poison—fear—
revolver—illness—doctor—brutal—marriage—too late." The
word "fear" is repeated three times. Round about the tomb-

stone are the words "guilt—fear—death—madness—end." All
these words indicate the patient's complexes, and therefore
provided important hints and starting-points for their discussion and interpretation. One can, for instance, guess from the
position and the special colouring of the word "father," that
the patient's relation to her father played a particularly important rôle. It was in fact just this strong negative father-
fixation which had caused a great deal of her neurotic troubles.
It is obvious that the drawing as a whole is the expression of a
depressed and negativistic state of mind; and the patient produced the picture in order to convince me that it was hope-
less to expect a cure. As a matter of fact, such a drawing might
well arouse doubts as to whether the patient's destructive forces
were not after all too strong. But, oddly enough, and very
fortunately, the patient's unconscious itself played a trick on
her and gave direct proof in the drawing that this was not so.
If one looks more closely at the central grave, one can see a
very remarkable sign of life which does not fit in at all with the
rest of the picture, namely a red-yellow-green circle. It is like
a kind of life-germ, which gives us, in spite of all negativity
of the remainder of the drawing, some proof of what one might
call the patient's capacity for psychic growth. As a matter of
fact, this circle is the first fragmentary emergence of a mandala.

It is characteristic that this germ of life is hidden in the
depth of the coffin, right down in the earth, symbolizing the
unconscious out of which future development will spring forth.
This drawing seems to me so particularly important and interesting, because it provides patent evidence in refutation of the
theory that such drawings are made artificially or are mere chance
products. For the one component of it which is the most decisive
was produced not only without any conscious intention on the
part of the patient but even in opposition to her conscious expectations.

The motive of the first picture is amplified in a second one,
which the patient drew a fortnight later (cf. picture 5, page 104).
This picture is divided into two parts by a black cross-beam. On

the cross-beam are written the words: "Warning—Danger of death," the meaning of which is repeated and intensified by the great padlock and the words "Entrance prohibited." Above the black cross-beam is a kind of storm scenery, with high waves, lightnings, black clouds and several S.O.S. signals; a ship is at the mercy of the stormy sea. But underneath the two warnings a completely different landscape becomes visible. There you find, for instance, the picture of a blossoming tree, and a number of other symbols, mostly positive in character, such as the stork with a baby in its beak, the hearts and so on. Right at the bottom there is a sort of psychological pedigree, showing on the left hand side the words: "Mother—grandmother—grandfather," and on the right hand side: "Father—grandmother—grandfather." It is significant that the mother's side on the left is characterized as positive by gay colours, while the father's side on the right shows mostly dark negative colours. This explains also some of the symbols on the right hand side which apparently belongs to the father. There is the square full of section-marks, symbolizing the legalistic unsympathetic mind of the father, or the chess-board with the words "check to the queen." On the other hand, the left side, the mother's side, contains only positive symbols. The shield of David, with the snake, the emblem of Aesculapius, symbolizes the analyst and therefore also analysis, and apparently this snake is doing its best to penetrate the barrier by spitting fire (libido) against it.

Obviously these symbols (as well as the significant words of the first picture) form a starting-point for a discussion of the pictures. The general meaning of the second picture might be formulated thus: the scenery above the cross-beam represents the conscious situation of the patient: floating about and almost completely at the mercy of a terrible doom. That is the situation which makes her send out an S.O.S., crying for help. The "Uranus" on the right hand side of the top part symbolized to the patient something like a personal guidance or a kind of light of hope in the midst of despair. The lower half of the picture, however, represents her unconscious situation, which looks much more hopeful. Perhaps one might even say that the germ of the first picture reappears in the symbol of the blossoming tree in a much more developed state; in any case germ and tree have exactly the same colours. The notice-boards and ghostly faces which we can see between the two scenes represent the patient's resistance to acknowledging the positive and progressive tendencies of her unconscious. Obviously enough, it is the first task of analytical treatment to break through these resistances, and this is aptly symbolized by the snake on the left hand side.

An interesting coincidence with this drawing is provided by a dream which the patient dreamed the following night. In it, she feels sick, as if she is just waking up from a narcosis. Then she is waiting in an ante-room to see Dr. Jung. She enters a room; there a woman performs a beautiful dance, overcoming certain attempts at interference. Then she is told to go and sleep in peace as she will be released the next morning. This dream sums up what has happened. She is waking up from her unconscious condition, and is now prepared to meet the "wise old man" in herself. Attempts at interference with her own feminine self-expression can now successfully be dealt with, and her freedom in the near future seems assured.

In her later drawings, the patient expressed very clearly this process of release and integration, which brought her into touch with the healing powers of her own unconscious. This is borne out by the third picture (about the twentieth she did altogether) which was made two months after the first two, and which shows clearly the amount of progress made by her analysis (cf. picture 2, page 33). This picture, which the patient herself entitled "The Singing Tree" has a completely different character from the two previous ones. The lowering, menacing and negative atmosphere has been replaced by a bright and gay and obviously positive mood. The tree, which in the second picture is indicated in a tentative and rather cryptic manner in the realm of the unconscious, has now definitely entered the realm of consciousness. The colours of the picture indicate a feeling of happiness and a willing acceptance of emotional life. If one compares this pic-

ture with the first ones, one will be able to gain some idea of
what such a picture can mean to a patient in this situation, and
how it may help her to realize the strength of her own positive
forces. It is also rather interesting to notice how greatly the
technical ability of the patient, which at first was rather slight,
has increased.

I want to discuss one more picture of this patient which is
among the last she did (cf. picture 6, page 105). It grew out of a
dream which she dreamed just two years after the start of her
analysis and which marked the end of it. Her dream was as follows: "I had been for a long while a passenger on an ocean-going
vessel and was getting very anxious to set foot on land once more.
On the tender which was to bring us into port I met an astrologer
and wanted to consult him about my horoscope. He spread this
out in front of me, and it resembled a stained glass window in a
church through which the sun was shining." This dream made
a vivid impression on my patient.

It is obvious that it points towards the end of her analysis,
which is symbolized by the voyage across the ocean—across the
deep waters of the unconscious. She feels that now she has to
"disembark," and take up her "land existence," her ordinary
life, once more. This is quite naturally a critical point, as
it means for one thing leaving the guidance of analysis and the
analyst behind her, and for another thing that all she has
experienced and learned on this voyage will now be put to the
acid test. So far her dream is a kind of *"rite de sortie."* The
second part seems to be, on the other hand, a *"rite d'entrée"*—
an attempt of her unconscious to define the position reached so
far, and to provide her with a kind of map for the future. The
figure of the astrologer would represent the archetype of the
"wise old man," the animus with some sort of superior esoteric
knowledge. The "horoscope" would be a symbol of the fateful
combination of her inborn character and problems. The church
window in the form of which the horoscope appears tends to
show that the dissociations in her earlier life, which brought
her to analysis, have been knitted together into a harmonious

whole. The sun shining through it might be taken as a kind of higher consciousness illuminating the pattern of her life.

It is not surprising that when she told me the dream, she felt that her words gave only an incomplete description of it; so much so that she felt she must give a more adequate expression of the salient feature of the dream, i.e. the horoscope or church window. The picture she drew is clearly of the mandala type, which Jung has described in *The Secret of the Golden Flower*,[1] and of which he has given numerous instances in *The Integration of the Personality*. It is a symbol of individuation as a representation of psychic entity or wholeness. The painting is a typical mandala, since it shows the central square and the surrounding circle. The square, with its reference to the number four, appears in all Eastern mandalas as "the courtyard of the monastery," with the four gates of consciousness— the wholeness of the four psychic functions; the circle is the "temenos," or the alchemical "krater," inside which the transmutation, "the opus alchymicum," that is the process of individuation, takes place.

The number six which appears in this mandala is also typical of Eastern ritual mandalas,[2] and is connected with the idea of the horoscope which is expressed in the dream.[3] The whole drawing points in symbolical form to the unity and integration of personality and it is clear how much this representation of psychological wholeness must mean—quite apart from its general significance—to a patient whose original problem had been that of a strong dissociation of her personality. It gives an idea as to why and how people come to think of drawing at all and what form such a symbolic expression of a dream content may take.

The last picture and the dream which preceded it are good examples of a case in which we can and indeed must enlarge the

[1] Richard Wilhelm and C. G. Jung: *The Secret of the Golden Flower*. Kegan Paul, London, 1931.
[2] Cf. the Tibetan mandala which Jung gives in *Psychologie und Alchemie*, Rascher, Zürich, 1944, p. 143.
[3] As a parallel cf. the Mexican Calendar in *Psychologie und Alchemie*, p. 149.

associations of the dreamer by our own knowledge. Jung has called this method of interpretation "amplification."[1] In it the original material—whether it be a dream or a drawing—is enriched by means of analogous images from mythology, folklore, etc. It is obvious that the very far-reaching archetypal symbolism which the material contains must of necessity be out of the dreamer's reach, and therefore she cannot understand the meaning of her drawing. It goes without saying that in such a case the analyst very often does not give the patient a detailed explanation of all the allusions and associations of the symbolism shown in his picture, but goes only as far as is necessary to make him understand the general meaning of it. It is not necessary to discuss all the theoretical material, but only that part of it which is indispensable for the understanding of the actual and acute situation of the patient. At a later stage of the analytical process, however, when the neurotic material has given place to the emergence of undistorted images of the collective unconscious, general discussion of this kind becomes more and more advisable and helpful. As to the question of the technical ability with which such a picture is done, we may say that it is relatively irrelevant; what really matters is the libido invested in its execution and the psychological and symbolical meaning which the picture possesses for its author. These pictures exert a singular effect on the dreamer, an influence so powerful that it appears almost magical. Looked at from the rational standpoint of everyday life, such pictures may appear more or less absurd; but experience shows that they possess a strongly constructive influence. The very fact that they originate in the unconscious gives them the power to compel the unconscious to give up its fascinating and compulsive hold upon the patient, and instead to set free its latent progressive energy.

An illustration of this, and also of the fact that this type of drawing does not require any artistic or pictorial skill in the patient, is provided by the drawings of a woman of thirty-eight who consulted me on account of marked agoraphobia. In

[1] Cf. Jung, *The Integration of the Personality,* p. 207.

the course of the analysis, she began quite spontaneously to form imaginative pictures of her condition, and a little later she proceeded to put these on paper. On page 74 are a few examples of the sequence of pictures which she produced in a few weeks. Apart from one picture (which is not given here), they all have as their subject the release of a suspended feminine figure from its enveloping shackles. At first this figure hung quite limp and motionless; then it began to move and struggle, until finally she sat free of her shackles in an easy-chair. Of this gradual development only the first two and the last two drawings are here reproduced. (Before the last two—on the threshold of freedom—she drew a picture of an opening door leading to a blossoming garden.) Complete restoration to health required, of course, a very much longer time, but the important fact is that such drawings contribute very largely to liberating the healing powers contained in the patient's unconscious. Not only are they a clear formulation of her situation, which helps her to realize much more consciously than ever before what the actual position is, but also they help to constellate the creative aspect of the unconscious. In the case of the woman suffering from agoraphobia, who had so long been a helpless victim to severe anxiety attacks, these pictures meant new hope and life, and thus helped to break the vicious circle of her neurosis.

*   *   *

In order to appreciate fully the value and function of such drawings, it is necessary to have observed the truly explosive effect which they often exert on the patients themselves. They derive that effect from their function as transformers of energy, as every other true symbol does. The level of symbolical representation in the mandala of the first woman on the one hand, and the drawings of the case of agoraphobia on the other hand, is obviously different. In the first case, we have a truly symbolical formulation of an experience that could not have been expressed equally adequately in any other way, whereas in the second case, on the surface no more is actually expressed than

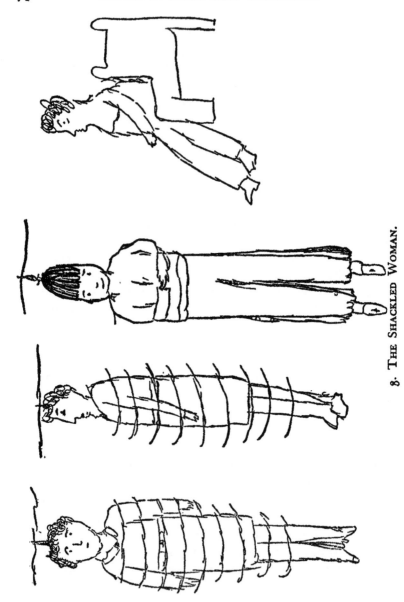

8. THE SHACKLED WOMAN.

might have been said in words. In other words: the mandala is a symbolical expression on the archetypal level, whereas the second series of drawings merely anticipates the release from neurotic symptoms. Nevertheless, the second series of drawings has symbolical value, because it helps to constellate energy that could not have been constellated otherwise. In this sense, such pictures—the mandala as well as those of the case of agoraphobia—act as an instrument of contemplation. They are what Indian psychology would call a "yantra,"[1] the means of activating, concentrating and containing energy from the unconscious.[2]

Another reason, and a very practical one, for encouraging the desire of our patients to draw, is that we are all of us only too much inclined to minimize the reality of our inner life, as opposed to the experiences of our external life. In other words, when a patient describes ideas arising from his unconscious, which very often do not fit into his conscious scheme of things, he is only too apt to look on such ideas as "nothing more than idle dreams," and does his best to forget them as quickly as possible. Indeed, since a neurosis consists in a dissociation of the component parts of a personality, the same negative forces which prevent a synthesis of these separated elements seek also to minimize the compensating effort made by the unconscious to bridge the gap. That is, the critical and sceptical faculties of our reluctant conscious mind seek, by a process of attenuation, to dissipate the reality of our inner experiences, until they are rendered almost imperceptible. But contents of the mind which have been clothed in outward form, even if "only" that of a drawing, cannot be denied reality; they have been given concrete shape, and can no longer be completely ignored by our

[1] Cf. Jung, *Psychologie und Alchemie*, p. 141.
[2] Cf. Hastings, *Encyclopaedia of Religion and Ethics*, Vol. III, p. 445 ab. (Article: Charms and Amulets (Indian)), where the Indian definition of the yantra is given as "that which holds, restrains, fastens." The article goes on to say that a yantra is "a combination of mystical symbols and diagrams . . . supposed to possess occult powers." The psychological explanation of these "occult powers" is given by the otherwise seemingly inexplicable influx of unconscious energy which does work what appears to be a miracle.

everyday consciousness. Even where this tendency towards minimizing the unconscious images has been overcome, these pictures still help one to hold on to an inner experience which is only too easily blurred by the strength of external facts. They give more substance to an experience which otherwise may tend to elude our grasp and to evaporate because of its strangeness and its remoteness from everyday life.

One more example may show how different ways of active imagination may be used together. It is the case of a man of thirty-five, a scientist of great intelligence. He was a one-sided extravert, highly intellectual and remarkably intuitive, that is, his intellect and his intuition represented his main and his auxiliary functions, whereas his feeling and sensation functions were both inferior, and so was his introverted side.

He consulted me in a state of depression, which had been brought about, as he explained, because he felt quite unable to concentrate, or indeed to do any work at all. He had the characteristic feeling that all his energies were simply melting away under his hands and disappearing into dark unspecified regions. This state of affairs threatened to undermine his whole existence. From his dreams, from which I shall quote a characteristic example, it was obvious that his unconscious was absorbing a quite unjustifiable amount of energy, which he could therefore no longer use for his conscious everyday life.

One of his first dreams was this: "My wife bought herself a hat and coat for £100," to which he immediately added, with obvious disapproval, that his wife would never really do such a thing as she was in real life a very unassuming woman. Such a dream could, of course, form the starting point for a long chain of free associations, and any material thus revealed might be of greater or lesser significance. If our objective is to discover the complexes of a patient from such a dream, we might unhesitatingly proceed along this path. If, however, our main interest is concentrated on the content of the dream as such, our interpretation will take a different course. Then we shall try to find out what significance the component parts of the dream have for the dreamer. Thus we may discover the meaning of the dream, and find out what it is that his unconscious is trying to convey to him through his dream as a compensation for the actual concrete situation in which he finds himself. His associations, which correspond to what are called above "controlled" or "circular" associations, give the following picture of the situation. His wife was actually, as he had said, a "very unassuming woman." He felt very dependent on her, so much so that he "would not know what to do without her." He felt "so tremendously taken up with external facts" that she formed an essential counterpoise "as her inner life was so strongly developed. This meant that he projected on to his wife his own inferior introversion, in other words that she had to carry his anima-projection. The hat he felt to symbolize an individual attitude, as the choice of hats was so characteristic for the individuality of a person. The coat he understood as "protection and external covering."

If we consider the dream as a whole, we can now understand its meaning: "My anima is using up a great deal more libido than I like or indeed than I am aware of, in order to produce a new individual and collective attitude." In this way, we have unearthed not the dreamer's "complexes" but the meaning of the dream, which tells him that his old exaggerated extraverted attitude was goading his unconscious into rebellion. Consequently, the latter was using up too much of his libido— a state of things which he had first to accept and then come to terms with, if his nervous instability was to be readjusted.

This point is important for various reasons. From the point of view of the patient, the antidote seemed to be to remove his disabilities by means of concentration exercises, suggestion, etc. But that would have meant to stimulate still more his extraverted side and would therefore in the long run undoubtedly have increased his state of tension to an even more unbearable degree. The right way from the analytical point of view is for him to aim at bringing about a better balance by yielding to the tendency to introversion which his unconscious was actually trying to force on him. For this man had quite obviously been letting his extraversion assume tyrannical dimensions, and his unconscious had reacted forcefully to this one-sidedness. This case illustrates once more the necessity of examining symptoms for their positive tendencies.

There could be no two opinions as to the necessity for this man to come somehow or other into constructive contact with his unconscious. Although it is unquestionably difficult for an intellectual and extraverted person to be willing to focus his attention on his unconscious processes and images, we were nevertheless able to find a way. My patient had mentioned that he was very fond of scribbling, and, as is well known, this is often with intellectual people a favourite mode of expression for the unconscious. I suggested therefore that he should cultivate his faculty in this line: he should sit down one evening at home and quite definitely and consciously allow this faculty free play. The result was a complete surprise and confirmed how great had been his need for a channel through which his unconscious could find its way to the daylight. At the next interview he brought me four sheets covered with "doodles," of which I shall select two for discussion, since the patient himself considered them specially significant.

Looked at rationally, these pictures seem rather absurd. In the first sketch (cf. p. 79, No. 1) two figures, in which the patient thought to recognize himself and his wife, are climbing a hill, but underneath them is a cave containing a series of remarkable symbols. The hatching at the bottom left-hand side represented, according to the patient, a kind of heap of undifferentiated primeval matter, forming a matrix from which the other objects in the cavern developed. This "undifferentiated primeval matter" is apparently what the alchemists would have called "materia prima," in which "the precious substance is potentially contained . . . in the form of a massa confusa."[1] In addition the cave contains a kind of fragmentary coat of arms, a crucifix and a crystal. The incomplete coat of arms indicates that the

[1] Jung, *The Integration of the Personality*, p. 245.

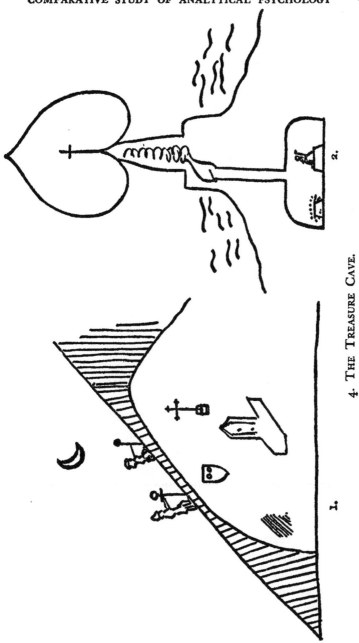

4. THE TREASURE CAVE.

process of development of the personality is still incomplete, and that, as is natural at his time of life, only about half of his personality had been formed. (The two dots represent half of the complete number of the four functions in particular, and of the four as a symbol of integration in general.) Crystalline structures were of frequent occurrence in the patient's subsequent drawings. This I took to point to a kind of process of crystallization and centralization in his unconscious, directed towards its end result, the crystal or philosopher's stone, symbolizing his integrated personality. But it was the crucifix which excited the patient most deeply. It seemed to him a clear indication that some kind of religious and irrational process in his unconscious was taking place, the alarming repercussions of which were flowing over into his conscious mind. As a matter of fact, the patient here came up against the very heart of his neurosis. The years round about thirty-five are, as is well known, very often a critical age in psychological development. It is as if at this middle point in our life we begin to get ready for a decisive change-over to another side of life to which justice must somehow be done if we are not to fall into a barren one-sidedness. This was quite obviously so in his case.

The dormant tendency to introversion and the need for a fuller integration of his personality which existed in his unconscious and demanded recognition and realization were largely responsible for his present conflict and found expression in these drawings. This is also hinted at by the moon, which shows that this is a nocturnal landscape, implying that the drawing symbolizes an excursion into the region of the unconscious. The meaning of the drawing as a whole is therefore: the patient finds himself in the company of his anima (=wife), who is the mediator between him and the deep layers of the psyche, on a difficult journey through the moon-landscape of the collective unconscious. In the course of this journey he comes to a treasure cave, concealing a number of mysterious symbols. It will apparently be his task to discover the meaning of these symbols, all of which refer to certain non-rational and integrative, that is in the widest sense "religious," tendencies in himself of whose existence he has hitherto been unaware. (Interesting in this connection is the peculiar shape of the staff in the hand of one of the figures. This bears a definite resemblance to a "crux ansata," the ancient Egyptian symbol of eternal life.) The drawing explains clearly why the patient is unable to concentrate, and has lost his energy. His libido is obviously enclosed within the symbols of the treasure-cave, where it must be sought, re-discovered and reconquered.

The next drawing (cf. p. 79, No. 2) shows how the patient has progressed on his journey in this direction. It represents a cavern under water; that is, psychologically speaking, the action is taking place in the depths of the collective unconscious, and is evidently very intense, to judge by the steam rising from a kind of chimney. The figures, or rather the dots, shown on the left-hand side of the cave, represent, as the patient, curiously enough, knew with complete certainty and had no hesitation whatsoever in stating, the Last Supper; whereas the figure on the right, according to him, represents a divine being, sitting on a throne.

There is a very good reason why the patient hits upon the symbol of the Last Supper. When acting with our fully differentiated functions and capacities, we are so self-reliant and self-satisfied that, as long as we can maintain our life on this level, we do not need the help of anyone. As soon as we are forced, however, to face our undeveloped and inferior side—our shadow—we are helpless in the grip of our limitations. Then we feel dependent and forlorn, and we experience for the first time what real loneliness may mean. But for this very reason it is only then that we begin to be truly human, and to come into contact with the real mystery of existence. This crisis of the undeveloped inferior side of our nature is frequently one of the necessary concomitants of the crucial turning-point in the middle of life. That which was formerly important becomes relatively unimportant and vice versa. That is why my patient, as soon as he became aware of his vulnerable spot, conceived the symbol of the Last Supper, with its profound significance of death and resurrection, and moreover the prototype of communion, of spiritual unity and fellowship. From this starting-point he may reach and realize an entirely new plane of existence. The need engendered by the patient's one-sided development and the cul-de-sac into which it had led him, called forth quite unexpected help from hitherto unknown levels. This is also illustrated by the symbol of the heart containing a cross. The image of the Last Supper, the communion between God and man, sets free energy which streams up from the layer of the collective unconscious into his personal life, creating in him the possibility of spiritualized feeling. This is another proof that a man needs to assimilate the opposite pole to his conscious personality, and this is the task required of the patient at this particular juncture of his life. Here and nowhere else he regains access to his "lost energies."

When we first discussed these pictures, my patient's reaction was remarkable. As we were looking at the pictures together, he suddenly flushed scarlet and began to weep. His unconscious had definitely reacted, and at the sight of his own drawings he had, at least for one instant, penetrated through the thin crust covering the cave. In this case it seemed desirable to strengthen his contact with the images of his unconscious, and I therefore proposed that he should set out on the way of active imagination in its strict sense, and foster his contact with this inner world of symbols. I suggested that he should spend some time in the evenings quite still and relaxed with closed eyes, and see if any pictures would emerge before his inner vision. My patient very quickly learned to catch his inner processes at work, and experienced quite definite relief and relaxation from this compensation for his outer unrest and worry. I should like to quote an example from the series of phantasies produced in this way which will demonstrate how closely drawing and imagination worked in the same direction.

Religious symbolism had occupied a strikingly central position in his pictures; and his phantasies confirm the fact that his neurosis was largely due to the repression of such deep-seated non-rational needs of his nature, which he had never previously allowed to come to life. While allowing his creative imagination free rein, my patient found himself wandering through a certain landscape. There he saw some distance away a little hut, towards which he walked. When he came nearer, he noticed that it was an earth-hut, and that there was a mysterious old woman inside. It is significant, as showing the absolute autonomous nature of such unconscious pictures, that he was unable, in spite of the greatest effort, to recognize the face of the woman.[1] A bright fire burns inside the hut and there is a strong and pleasant smell of food. The old woman asks him if he would like some soup, and since he is very hungry, he is delighted at the invitation. He sits down inside the hut at a table which is made of a slab of slate supported by four stones. Suddenly he finds a piece of chalk between his fingers and he knows that he has got to make a drawing on the table. While he is sitting wondering what to draw, there suddenly appears to him in a vision (i.e. a vision in a vision, which indicates that a deep layer of the unconscious has been reached), a vivid procession of "holy people" walking in the air. First comes Christ in white robes, then Mahomet, followed by "a group of people of the same kind." Then he knows in a flash what he has to draw, or as he characteristically puts it in his phantasy, "what I am supposed to draw," namely "the ripple interference pattern which you get when throwing a stone into a pond—ripples drawn with a concentric pattern going out into infinity." Then the vision ends thus: "Lovely flower in front of me—green leaves and fresh salmon pink petals go out in concentric circles."

The gist of the phantasy is sufficiently self-evident. It runs more or less parallel with the symbolism of the two drawings, only that it embodies the answer to his psychological problem in a more definite symbol. The woman of the phantasy is again an anima figure, but now separated from his wife—that is, the

---

[1]This fact is important as an answer to the objection that these phantasies are produced by our conscious will. But the only use we make of our conscious will is to focus on a psychic background which is usually completely unconscious. Thus we do not produce these pictures, but give them a chance to come up and act upon us.

projection on to her has been withdrawn. She is the "wise old woman," the feminine counterpart of the figure of the "wise old man," which invites him into her magic circle and nourishes him. The vision of religious figures brings him face to face with his neglected inner reality, and this is finally summed up in the beautiful symbol of the ripple-interference pattern. Here his unconscious has provided him with a personal religious experience of a universal symbol. It shows a movement going out from a centre, a middle point, a symbol which actually represents the exact opposite to his way of life, where the centre had been missing, so that in consequence he had been identified with everything outside himself. This interference pattern is a pointer towards the mandala symbol, which finally takes shape in the beautiful flower. At the same time, this is an interesting and instructive example of how an action may be transformed into a symbolical pattern: the procession of religious figures, a symbolical expression of a new order of his life, appears transformed into the symbol of the mandala.

The effect of such inner processes is considerable. It would be one thing if I had tried to explain to my patient a psychological fact, but it is quite a different thing if he has to face the identical fact from inside as experienced in his own phantasy. For it is a layer of his own psyche—an "inner voice"—which is talking to him; it is his experience and is therefore much more genuine and effective than if it had been an idea coming from another person. The most important feature, of course, is the activation of the patient's own healing tendencies. Therefore our task consists in helping the patient to seize these images and symbols and in explaining to him their meaning, and so assisting him to make conscious use of them for the actual and acute situation in which he finds himself.

I have just described the two chief methods used in the technical application of active imagination; but for the sake of completeness, I must add that there exists a whole series of other possibilities. It is possible, for instance, for a patient to make use of modelling instead of drawing; and sometimes our patients

invent the oddest means of expressing the contents of their unconscious, in which case it is obviously best to let them go their
own way. Another possibility is, for instance, that mentioned
before of an inner dialogue with figures of a dream or phantasy,
that is with the personified contents of the unconscious.

In conclusion, I should like to emphasize the fact that the
method of active imagination can and should only be used by
those psychotherapists who have themselves experienced it; just
as it is a sine qua non for an analyst of whatever school to
have been analysed himself. Moreover, this technique can only
be employed and accepted in its full implications when it is
based on a definite attitude on the part of the analyst, namely
when he himself is absolutely convinced of the creative validity
of the contents of the unconscious. For the unconscious is not a
dustbin in which one finds all the cast-off and indigestible contents of the mind, but on the contrary, it is the matrix of the
conscious mind. It is only on this basis that the method of
active imagination can be understood. Only when a neurosis is
conceived as the ultima ratio of the psyche, which is making
in this way a supreme and valiant effort to force on the patient
the realization of the suppressed but potentially constructive
elements in his own mind, can we take the great responsibility
of encouraging a patient to surrender so completely to the
images of his unconscious. Indeed, the use of these methods
merely as a superficial technique may lead to serious damage
to the patient, for obviously there is a danger that the unconscious may get the upper hand unless the strictest control is
exercised by the analyst, amounting at times to actual pro-
hibition of further imaginings.

Just because the examples of active imagination which have
been discussed so far show all the positive possibilities, some of
the dangers that lurk in meeting one's unconscious at such close
quarters have also to be mentioned. In describing the case of the
man of thirty-five, and discussing his drawing of the treasure-
cave, I said that the patient with the help of his phantasy had
penetrated through the thin crust which covered the cave into

its interior. But this process of penetration through the crust can sometimes lead to a sudden fall into an abyss, and such a breaking through may cause drowning or produce an explosion; indeed in extreme cases the force of the impact may rupture the thin skin which is mercifully covering a latent psychosis. Such a situation calls for the greatest care and experience on the part of the analyst. In any case, there must be careful timing, for contents of the unconscious which can be assimilated by the conscious mind if it is sufficiently integrated by the analytical process and if the relationship with the analyst is sufficiently strong, can have the most destructive effect in a case where these premises do not exist. We must never forget to include in our calculations the very relative factor of the stability of the conscious mind, for in the last resort it is always the ego, the centre of the conscious personality, which has to fulfil the task of integration. Thus, for instance, I remember a case where I was reminded of this factor in a very unpleasant manner. I had told a patient to continue drawing her phantasies at home. A few hours later she rang me up in a thoroughly desperate state: picture after picture was rushing at her, and she felt completely powerless to resist the force of the images coming up from the unconscious. I had to see her at once in order to stop this state which represented, so to speak, an artificially induced psychosis. It is on such occasions that the vital importance of the personal contact between analyst and patient becomes particularly obvious. Without this strong and safe contact the situation might have become desperate.

I should like to illustrate this by another picture (cf. picture 7, page 120). It is the drawing of a woman of about forty. A globe is just on the point of falling into an abyss. If one gets such a drawing one cannot be too careful. Such a situation as is expressed in this picture lays upon us the obligation to refrain for the time being from all attempts at analysis. The only thing we can do is to stand by as a potential source of help while a process whose course is at present more or less unalterable unrolls itself. But nevertheless, such a case is, in the long run, not necessarily beyond our reach. As a matter of fact, even such a seemingly disastrous drawing may conceal certain positive features. If the patient realizes the meaning of the situation as it is expressed in the picture, the situation may be transformed. At present she is more or less pushed into the abyss; but this movement downwards into the unconscious must correspond to a deep necessity of her psychological situation. She is obviously "too high up" and has therefore to "go down." If she can accept this downward movement, the fall into the abyss might be transformed into a "katabasis eis antron,"[1] the "descent into the cave" of the unconscious, as a compensation for a too exalted conscious position. (The patient was actually a woman of great intellectual powers and her feeling side was definitely inferior.) The question is always how much of the unconscious problem can be integrated, and in this the decisive factor is how firmly the ego is established.

This more hopeful possibility is borne out by two pictures which the same patient drew later, after a previous state of severe depression had come to an end (cf. picture 8, page 121). The first picture is that of a blossoming tulip, the growth of which is seriously hampered by a black ring. The flower cannot unfold, and only through death is it freed from the ring. This is obviously the representation of a neurotic depression, which interferes in a fatal manner with the emotional life of the patient. Therefore the next drawing is important, for in it the ring has disappeared, and, instead of the dying flower, one sees a widely opened flower which, in the original colours, looks almost like an oil lamp with a golden flame or a receptacle of light.

Activation of the unconscious may also be to a certain extent limited by the type structure of the patient. Thus it is often more difficult for an extravert than for an introvert to face the pictures of his unconscious, and particularly so when the extraversion is allied to a strong sensation type. (In the case quoted of the strongly extraverted man, his intuition was a definite

[1] Cf. Jung, *Psychologie und Alchemie*, p. 450; *The Integration of the Personality*, p. 150.

help to active imagination.) Just as it is clearly necessary to proceed more carefully and to tread more delicately when trying to adjust an introvert to the necessities of the outer world than would be the case with an extravert, the same holds good when dealing with an extravert and the requirements of his inner world.

This reminds me of a woman patient of mine, a very one-sided extravert, belonging to the sensation type, who had landed herself in serious difficulties because of the expansive character of her emotional life. She had already been analysed for several months when she related a fragmentary dream which caused me to urge her to develop the dream situation by using active imagination. In her dream, she had seen a room, the back wall of which was entirely covered with shelves closed in by curtains. I asked her to shut her eyes and tell me what she could see in the room. It was the first time that I had asked her to do anything of the sort, and my patient, who for all these months had been patiently and bravely telling me about and discussing the most trying things, was quite unable to keep her eyes shut even for ten seconds. She was constantly opening them and protesting against the violence I was doing her. And indeed from her point of view, with perfect propriety, because the life of an extravert is so bound up with the outer world that if he is made to look within he may feel as if he were confronted almost with chaos.

However, she finally succeeded in her efforts and thereupon she discovered that the curtains had been drawn back and that thousands of books were standing on the shelves. A man entered the room, climbed up a ladder and rummaged violently about among the books, so much that a whole heap of them fell on his head and knocked him off his ladder. Again and again the man climbed up the ladder and ransacked the shelves, and again and again he was knocked off the ladder. This phantasy is a striking expression of the patient's heedless way of life, through which she—or, as one might also put it, her negative animus—had produced all the disorder and failures which had finally brought her to me. Thus this phantasy was quite useful from the point of view of therapy. When at last I put a stop to this rather cruel game (which from start to finish did not take more than five minutes), my patient was completely exhausted and very seriously annoyed with me. This is a harmless example, but it shows how differently different psychological types will react to such things in given circumstances and how these factors must be taken into consideration, at any rate when assessing tempo and dosage.

To sum up, it must be emphasized that active imagination must not be considered as a panacea. There exist cases when its use would be too dangerous; some patients cannot adopt the right frame of mind towards it, and it is always a mistake to try to force any method of dealing with the unconscious on anyone. Moreover, its use should, generally speaking, be restricted to the later stages of the analysis, when phantasies of the kind illustrated above often begin to occupy the place formerly taken by dreams, over which they have in general the merit of greater clearness, concentration and intensity. And finally: as with the passage of time, such phantasies or drawings contain an increasing number of figures emanating from the collective unconscious—i.e. archetypes—a specialized knowledge of ethnology, mythology and the psychology of religion is required.

To conclude this discussion of the technique of Analytical Psychology, there should be added just one word on another fundamental problem inherent in any and every technique: namely, that no technique can or should possess universal validity, since every general technique must disregard not only the individuality of the patient but also another very decisive and unique factor in the case, that is, the individuality of the analyst. We all start with general rules, but in the end each of us will, during the course of his work, develop his own individual "technique." One man will adopt one method as being best suited to his own individuality, whereas another will find some other way more natural to him. It is scarcely necessary to point out how carefully we must guard against the possibility of forcing our own preferences and inclinations on our patients. This does not mean, however, that we have not each one of us certain capacities and limitations which will and must to some extent prescribe the particular methods we employ. For it is nonsense to suppose that we can ever completely cut out our own subjective personality. On the contrary, what matters is that we should use to the utmost the specific and individual powers in it by which we can help another person; and that means that we should know our "personal equation." This again shows how indispensable is the analysis of the psychotherapist himself.

This brings me to the most important limitation of every technique. Inevitably there comes a point in every analysis where "technique" loses its meaning. This point is always reached when we have to deal with the patient not as a sick person but simply as an individual in his own right. At that point the words "analyst" and "patient" lose their meaning, and analysis becomes a living argument between two equal partners. This means the revealing of the true personality of the analyst, and no technique can give him help or shelter at this point. The analyst turns from a "psychotherapist" into but one pole of a mutual psychological process, and accordingly he is just as much the one who receives as the one who gives. His whole human personality is challenged, for the human problems of the "patient" no longer represent "pathological phenomena" but ask for human answers and decisions on a plane common to both partners in the analytical relationship.

Analysis here becomes a "reciprocal interplay of two psychic systems."[1] In this dialectic relationship—as Jung has called it—"the physician must step out of his anonymity and give an account of himself, exactly as he demands of his patient."[2] Every flaw in the integrity of the analyst's personality will be shown up without mercy, and no analyst can really help a patient beyond the level of his own consciousness. This obviously re-

---

[1]Jung, *Grundsätzliches zur praktischen Psychotherapie, Zentralblatt für Psychotherapie und ihre Grenzgebiete*, Hirzel, Leipzig, Vol. VIII, Heft 2, p. 67.
[2]Ibid., p. 80.

quires the strictest self-education of the psychotherapist himself. The dialectical relationship "demands not only the transformation of the patient, but also the counter-application to himself by the doctor of the system which he prescribes in any given case. And in dealing with himself the doctor must display as much relentlessness, consistency and perseverance as in dealing with his patients."[1]

In the last resort the personality and integrity of the analyst is therefore infinitely more important than his "technique." "Technique" is the necessary beginning; but the deeper the analytical process goes, the more it widens out into natural and indefinable life.

[1]Jung, "Problems of Modern Psychotherapy," in: *Modern Man in Search of a Soul*, p. 59.

III

STUDY OF A DREAM

THE CONCEPT of the collective unconscious stands at the very centre of the theory of Analytical Psychology. According to this, certain psychic behaviour and reaction patterns lie hidden as potentialities behind and beneath the individual psyche of each particular human being. These potential patterns cannot be explained from the personal experiences of the individual, but are the psychic sediment deposited by the development of the human soul throughout its age-long history. This concept of the *collective unconscious,* together with its manifestations the *archetypes,* is undoubtedly Jung's greatest contribution to modern psychology. The world of the collective unconscious and of the archetypes is so rich and so protean in its manifestations that, except for those who have themselves passed through analytical experience, the subject is necessarily somewhat difficult of approach and understanding. This difficulty is indicated in the question so often levelled at Analytical Psychologists as to the practical use and therapeutic value of this concept of the collective unconscious and the archetypes. This essay is an attempt to answer this question. The distinctive mode of approach and special possibilities offered by Analytical Psychology are illustrated by the study of a dream. The value of this dream for purposes of demonstration is greatly enhanced by the fact that it set in motion a process known as *active imagination.* The discussion of this process will lead us still deeper into the problems opened up by the methods employed in Analytical Psychology.

The dream is that of a man of thirty, a lawyer, a one-sided intellectual, with intuition as an auxiliary function. He came for treatment suffering from a markedly negative mother-fixation. This fixation had worked itself out in an unusual way. As a youth of eighteen, the patient met a young girl at a dancing class, to whom he was violently attracted in spite of a complete lack of response on her part, so much so that she soon refused to meet him. The patient, however, did not give up his infatuation, but used it to build up an elaborate world of phantasy around her which completely prevented him from having any other contacts with the opposite sex. The dominant feature of this phantasy world was a belief which he accepted without any reservation that this girl and he were intended for one another by "fate," that she was merely trying to run away from this fact, and that in due course they would be united, even if it took years and years to accomplish. This conviction was in no way influenced by the fact, which he had known for several years, that the girl had already bound herself to another man. His thoughts and feelings continued no less to circle ceaselessly round her person. This condition finally reached such a pitch that he became subject to hallucinations and believed that he was constantly seeing her in the street or at a theatre or elsewhere; and he would pester her with letters which she strongly resented, whereupon he would fly into an ungovernable rage. These hallucinations and emotional outbursts reduced him to such a state that he finally decided to undergo an analysis. From his symptoms it was evident that the patient possessed in many respects a schizophrenic border-line personality, with dangerous disruptive tendencies. This fact must be borne in mind, and I shall revert to it at a later stage.

As to the analysis, this soon revealed the fact that except for their first meeting twelve years ago, his so-called love affair had no foundation in fact whatsoever. It was not based, as might well have been the case, on real affection felt for an actual person, but the girl was to all intents and purposes a creature of phantasy, functioning merely as a figure on which to project his emotions. The relation, therefore, was not the expression of genuine feeling but a symptom of his negative mother-fixation. For this had driven him into such violent opposition to everything connected with the opposite sex that he had built up an imaginary love relation in order to confirm and intensify this antagonism, and thus avoid ever really facing up to the genuine problems of love and the emotional side of life. His situation was very acute, and the first three months of the analysis were spent in discussing this and in unravelling the main threads of his elaborate system of infantile reaction. After three months of analysis the patient brought the following dream which is studied in this paper:

"I am present at a party which I find very boring. I pass into an adjoining room. There I see in a corner two toy animals with which I begin to play. One of the animals is an ordinary sized teddy bear, the other is a wolf. The wolf is about a quarter the size of the teddy bear, and his pads are furnished with very sharp claws. It occurs to me that these claws render him very life-like, and at the same time extremely dangerous, so that he should be firmly seized by the scruff of the neck. This I proceed to do in order to prevent him turning round and clawing me. Then I allow the wolf to claw the bear's fur, telling the latter that he need not be afraid as I will see to it that the wolf does him no harm. Suddenly the wolf escapes from under my hand. He immediately runs out of the room and out of the house, and I know that once outside he will quickly grow into a large and dangerous animal. Someone says that what I am here experiencing is the primeval worm, the giant serpent encircling the world, or, as might equally well be said, the dragon, the adversary of man."

The patient was very much impressed by this dream, although quite unable to furnish any associations. In order to set his unconscious reactions going, I suggested that he should try to make a picture of the "giant serpent encircling the world" and he promptly adopted my suggestion. Two days later, he brought me not only one drawing, but a series of five, and informed me that when he had finished painting the first picture he experienced an irresistible impulse to continue drawing, so much so that he spent the entire night making this series of pictures. He said they were quite spontaneous, and were drawn without any conscious volition or control on his part, as if indeed the pictures had drawn themselves, a condition typical of the processes of active imagination. It was only after he had completed the fifth picture that he experienced a sense of fulfilment and relief which allowed him to stop working. As for the meaning contained in the pictures, this was, if anything, even more of a riddle to him than the dream.

The patient could not supply associations either to the dream or to the pictures. From this we may conclude that the symbolism of the dream, as well as that of the pictures, originated in a psychic level beyond the ordinary reach of the dreamer's consciousness; that is, it does not contain personal contents, but rather archetypes, which are the manifestations of the collective unconscious. Faced with such a special situation, we are justified —in contradistinction to our usual practice of using the patient's associations—in intervening ourselves because of our knowledge of collective symbolism; indeed, such intervention on our part is essential if we wish to discover the meaning of such a content. I will, therefore, apply in the following interpretation our method of *amplification,* that is of making use of parallels drawn from mythology and folklore.

The dream may be divided into three episodes, as follows: (1) a party at which the dreamer is very bored; (2) an adjoining room in which he finds the animals—this forms the main action; (3) "outside," where the wolf changes into the primeval worm— the serpent—the dragon.

We look on dreams as "the spontaneous self-revelation in symbolical form of the actual state of the dreamer's unconscious."[1] Our main problem is always to discover what one-sided and therefore unsatisfactory attitude in conscious life is being *compensated* by the dream, because we believe that the relation of the unconscious to the conscious psyche is com-

---

[1] Jung, *Ueber die Energetik der Seele,* p. 157.

pensatory. Therefore a knowledge of the actual situation of the patient, as described earlier, is necessary. From the discussion of the dream with the patient the meaning of the *boring party* became clear, namely, that it revealed in the unconscious the compensatory factors to his sterile social attitude. A "party" may symbolize either that one is well adapted to social and communal life, or, on the other hand, that one is being submerged in it. A "party" also personifies everyday life, that is, the part of our life and psychology which is completely covered by the field of our ego complex, and hence it may symbolize the ego. The development of the ego consciousness is certainly an essential concomitant of every psychological advance, but it should not be achieved at the expense of the instinctive and natural powers of the individual. For the realm of the ego is only the top layer above a vast realm of unrealized unconscious contents which have to be assimilated as far as possible. A one-sided identification of the whole psyche with the ego complex, which after all only represents a part of the personality, would lead to an arbitrary restriction of the whole personality, and the repression by the ego of all those tendencies which it might conceive as possible sources of danger; moreover, it involves being cut off from all genuine emotional experience. No life is complete that is identified with the limited area of social life, or what one might call the collective consciousness; and therefore the comment made by the unconscious on the dreamer's one-sided attitude finds vivid expression in his condition of boredom. We find a situation boring if it offers us nothing new, or stimulating, or constructive. This is the dreamer's situation in his everyday life, which it is his duty to set about changing. The dream, however, does not rest content with mere criticism, it points the way to new and vital experiences.

At this juncture, we can with advantage make use of a fact discovered through long experience in the interpretation of dreams, namely that these can often be divided into three parts, corresponding to a *threefold chronological pattern* consisting of past, present and future. Our dream shows this threefold division very clearly; the party, the room adjoining and the outside. The party, therefore, states the original problem with which the patient starts, that is, the cause of his neurosis rooted in his past history; the subsequent step, when he enters the adjoining room, represents his present critical situation; that is, it states his present problem which is crying out for a solution, and we may assume that the third act which takes place "outside" foreshadows the future in which the patient may attain to a new insight and to a more mature attitude to life once his present acute difficulties have been overcome. The immediate and urgent need, therefore, is that the patient, convinced of the barrenness of his present completely one-sided attitude, with its resultant nervous disturbances, should make up his mind to take the next step. What does this further step imply? He moves out of the region of social boredom, and of his one-sided intellectualism, into the "adjoining room," which is empty, except for two toy animals, with which he begins to play. During this game, or rather, to give the dynamic potency of the dream its due, because of and through this game, the two playthings come to life. This coming alive occurs in play, as it were casually and almost inadvertently; for through "playing" with them the objects are supplied with psychic energy and life. Through playing the activity of phantasy is stimulated, and in this way new potentialities are created.[1]

[1]"Play" conveys first and foremost the idea of something done simply as a game, almost without intention and, as it were, by the way. But in addition to this, to play with something means to give oneself up to the object with which one plays; one so to speak infuses one's own libido into the thing played with. As a result of this the play develops into a magic action which conjures up life. It has long been known that the play of primitives and children represents a magic action which for them possesses absolute reality, though on a different level from so-called "concrete" reality. To play means to bridge over the gap between phantasy and reality by the magical action of one's own libido; play is thus a "rite d'entrée" which prepares the way for adaptation to the real object. This is why the play of primitives so easily passes over into earnest. It is reported of all kinds of primitive races that war games between two tribes readily "degenerate" into fights in which people are killed and wounded. Cf. for example Werner: *Einführung in die Entwicklungspsychologie*, Barth, Leipzig, 1926, p. 136ff.: "Just

It will be readily understood that animals in dreams represent the level of the instincts. An animal is "subhuman," and stands for the animal side of our nature; animals express the instinctual libido and, in general, the unconscious.[1] But why in particular a bear, a wolf and a snake? In order to answer this question in the absence of all associations on the part of the dreamer, it is necessary to draw on our knowledge of collective psychic material. To begin with the *bear*. From very ancient times the bear has been used as a symbol of motherhood. It plays a prominent rôle in Greek antiquity, and, choosing from an immense number of examples, I will confine myself to an account of a few specially characteristic ones. The bear plays an important part, for instance, in the cult of Artemis, the goddess most closely associated with the typical functions of the feminine sex: she is the tutelary deity of childbirth and is intimately concerned with the care of children. It was customary for young girls before marriage to bring her as votive offerings their tresses, or jewellery or playthings.[2] Artemis and her priestesses were often represented as she-bears; at an annual initiation ceremony in Athens little girls between five and ten years old performed symbolically the rites of the priestesses of Artemis; they were dressed in bearskins and were known as *arktoi* or the bears. This cult of the she-bear, referring particularly to the

---

as, for example, among one of the most primitive races known to us, the Veddas in Ceylon, battle scenes in games frequently lead to actual fights, so also an actual hunt or the catching of wild animals is immediately followed by the performance of the hunting play. (In the latter case the play acts in the contrary sense as a *"rite de sortie,"* by which the adaptation to the reality of every-day life is restored.) Even in the case of primitive peoples who are to some degree civilized it happens often enough that the spectators intervene in the action of a drama which is being performed just as if it were a reality, and sometimes the actor who is representing a villain is beaten on the stage. . . ."

The play of children has been called an act of "unintentional self-development" (Groos, quoted from C. W. Valentine, *The Psychology of Early Childhood*, Methuen, London, 1942, p. 150). It is an unconscious and instinctive preparation for later "serious" activities. In play we find reflected "the child's relation not only to inner events, but also to people and events in the outside world." (M. Fordham, *The Life of Childhood*, Kegan Paul, London, 1944, p. 110f.)

[1] Cf. Jung, *Modern Man in Search of a Soul*, p. 29.

[2] Preller-Robert, *Griechische Mythologie*, 4th edition, Weidmann, Berlin, 1894. Vol. I, p. 319.

ethical side of maternity, is found in all parts of the ancient world where the cult of the Magna Mater exists.

To mention another instance from quite a different quarter, we may recall the bear goddess Artio of Celtic origin, whose fame is probably perpetuated in the coat of arms of the Swiss town of Berne. Such examples could be multiplied at will. This symbolism is based on the well-known fact of natural history that bear cubs are particularly helpless young animals, and that she-bears are noted for the tender and self-sacrificing care they lavish on their young. In any case, ancient writers such as Pliny and Plutarch lay great stress on this characteristic, and there is no doubt that the she-bear is pre-eminently a mother symbol, a fact fully borne out by much psychological material.

The symbolism of the *wolf* is not quite so straightforward. To begin with, the wolf like the bear represents a mother symbol, but in this case the emphasis is chiefly laid on the maternal instinct as shown in care for the stranger and the outcast, that is, those who are in danger of destruction. The best-known example occurs in Roman mythology where the she-wolf suckles the twin founders of the Eternal City. It is, however, a remarkable fact that the wolf plays a very alarming and uncanny rôle in most other mythologies. Even in Rome the wolf did not always bear a benign aspect. Lupa, or she-wolf, was a common term for harlot, which is the exact antithesis of the maternal aspect of woman. This name for harlot obviously arises from the predatory nature of wolves. To Dante the wolf is the symbol of avarice and of the greed for material possessions.[1] In Greek mythology the wolf, that fierce denizen of dark and wintry forests, personifies devouring plagues, or the "pestilence that walketh in darkness,"[2] and is opposed by the god of light, Apollo, another name for whom is Lykios (from *lykos*, wolf), that is, the god who scares away the prowling wolf from the herds and flocks. In Nordic mythology the wolf plays an especially characteristic

[1] Cf. *Divina Commedia, Inferno* I, 49, *Purgatorio,* XX, 10.
[2] It is interesting that e.g. to the Red Indians of North America the wolf is the representative of the waning or dark moon; it is opposed to the power of light (cf. Krickeberg, *Indianermärchen aus Nordamerika,* Diederichs, Jena, 1924, p. 373).

part. He is the diabolical inhabitant of the wilderness, he is the Fiend. As such, he has the power of the evil eye. The sinister rôle of the wolf as "werewolf," or wolf-man, a shape much affected by sorcerers and witches, is well known. Echoes of this rôle can still be found in the fairytale of Red Riding Hood.

The strongest expression of the uncanny and destructive nature of the wolf is to be found in the Edda, in the saga of the Fenris wolf. The giantess Angreboda, harbinger of evil, bears to Loki the following three monsters who bring destruction on gods and men: Hel, the goddess of the underworld; Jörmungand, the serpent of Midgard, and most terrible of all the ruthless Fenris wolf. At the end of the world when gods and giants meet in mortal combat, it is the Fenris wolf who swallows the highest god Odin. Together with Hel and the Midgard serpent it is the dangerous adversary of the gods, and as such the symbol of the end of the world.[1] An interesting parallel to the events in our dream is afforded by the fact that in Nordic mythology, immediately after birth, the three monsters Hel, the Midgard serpent and the Fenris wolf rapidly grow to monstrous proportions, just as in the dream the wolf quickly grows into a large and dangerous animal. Another point of similarity is that in the dream the wolf appears closely related to the snake and to its equivalents the primeval worm and the dragon: this is another remarkable parallel to the Nordic myth in which the Fenris wolf and the Midgard serpent are brother and sister. The meaning of the wolf in the dream is clearly connected with its fierce and predatory nature; it represents the dark, uncanny principle of the underworld.

In order fully to grasp the symbolism of the bear, and even more especially of the wolf, one must keep in mind the latter's transformation into the snake. The *snake* is one of the most pregnant symbols of the unconscious, so much so that it often stands for the unconscious itself. Just as the symbolical im-

[1]The wolf plays a similar rôle in the Persian Avesta, where it is said that after the victory of Ahuramazda—the good principle—the time of the Wolf will have passed and that of the Lamb is to begin. (Cf. Chantepie de la Saussaye, *Lehrbuch der Religionsgeschichte*, Mohr, Tübingen, 1925, Vol. II, p. 253.)

portance of the bear is due to its elaborate care for its young
and that of the wolf is based on its fierce and predatory nature,
so in the case of the snake its symbolical meaning is due to
certain facts of natural history. Since snakes frequent underground caves and swamps, it has come to be considered a
chthonic earthbound animal, a divinity of the underworld; the
fact that it casts its skin gave rise to a belief in its immortality;
its secret and uncanny approach renders it symbolical of the
sinister power of the instincts, and indeed of the unconscious as a
whole, which works secretly in the dark but can strike with
lightning rapidity. Owing to its poisonous nature it stands for
daemonic power, as well as by an apotropaic reversal of rôles
as the healing serpent of Aesculapius. The snake, in its rôle of
god of the underworld and symbol of the earth, appears for
instance in Greek folklore as the giant Python, who personifies
the underworld and was slain by Apollo, the god of light, who,
to commemorate his victory, founded the temple of Pytho in
Delphi, with its ministering priestess Pythia.[1] The gloomy
character of the snake, the inhabitant of the underworld, ac-
counts for its use as a symbol of the Adversary who appears
in so many legends and sagas, e.g. the story of the Fall, the
Babylonian Tiamat, the Midgard serpent which also symbolizes
the Flood, and so on. The dragon, or the snake, appear frequently as guardians of the treasure lying hidden in the bowels
of the earth, which can only be recovered after the dragon is
slain. On the other hand, the conquest of the dragon or snake
confers peculiar power or wisdom, as can be seen by the name
given to the Greek priestess Pythia; or in the saga of Siegfried,
who defeats the dragon and drinks his blood and so is made
free of the language of the birds.[2] This is a symbolization of the

[1] The cult of the snake which is associated with the Erinnies, is also part of
their veneration as chthonic goddesses. With reference to Pythia cf. Hans Leisegang, *Die Gnosis*, Kröner, Leipzig, 1924, p. 111: "A dragon sends to Pythia from
the interior of the earth the pneuma which causes ecstasy, and she herself is
represented seated on the tripod with a snake on her knees." More examples can
be found e.g. in Erwin Rohde's *Psyche*.

[2] Cf. also the legend of Melampos, whose ears were purified while he slept by a
pair of serpents, after which he was able to understand the language of wood-

experience that man, by "overcoming," i.e. by integrating, the forces of the "underworld" (that is of the unconscious, instinctual powers), gains special knowledge. Another instance of this is the part played by the serpent in the Eleusinian mysteries of Demeter, during which the initiate had to kiss an artificial snake to symbolize his assimilation of the powers of the underworld.[1] Being cold-blooded, the snake also represents the cold, inhuman, unrelated aspect of the instincts, i.e. of the merely biological reflex actions; its sinister surprise attacks[2] and perilous nature make it, *par excellence,* a symbol of fear. The ceremony of kissing the snake during the celebration of the mysteries symbolizes, therefore, victory over this beast of fear; it represents the conquest and assimilation (=kiss) of man's dark instincts, thus bringing about their integration and the achievement of psychological redemption and completion.

We find a direct continuation of this symbolism in the early Christian Gnosticism, in particular in the practices of the gnostic sect of the Ophites. These celebrated the Eucharist by placing a collection of bread on a table and allowing a snake to writhe through the heaped-up bread. They then kissed the mouth of the snake and prostrated themselves in front of it. To them the snake, which they called "Naas" or "Ophis," is the symbol of the *nous,* the knowledge and wisdom that creates the world and vouchsafes redemption; so that to them the snake actually sym-

---

worms and birds (Bachofen, *Urreligion und antike Symbole* (ed. by C. A. Bernoulli), Reclam, Leipzig, 1926, Vol. 2, pp. 57, 439)—a particularly apt image of the unconscious as the bringer of wisdom. In Japanese mythology the hero Susanowo slays the giant snake, finds in it a miraculous sword, and marries the maiden whom he has saved from the snake. (Chantepie de la Saussaye, Vol. 1, p. 281f.)

[1]The remains of a great terracotta serpent were found at Eleusis (Preller, Vol. 1, p. 797, note 1). Demeter is the goddess of earth, and as mother of Persephone the goddess of the underworld.

[2]Its character of taking by surprise has led to the snake being given the significance of lightning, or of storm-wind and rain (cf. Danzel, *Mexico,* I, Folkwang, Hagen, 1923, pp. 38, 45) and of the flood (as in the Nordic myth in the form of the Midgard serpent; cf. Edda, Voluspa); it is thus also an image for the "lightning-like" and "overwhelming" character of the unconscious instinctual level (cf. Jung, *Psychology of the Unconscious,* Kegan Paul, London, 1921, pp. 266 and 333f.— footnote 61).

bolizes the Saviour himself. The belief in the hidden wisdom of the serpent is related to its use as a symbol for the dark, instinctual levels. That is why, for instance, the snake was chosen as the animal of Aesculapius, no doubt also because it carries poison; and snakes were kept in his temple in Epidauros.[1] From the point of view of psychology, it is interesting to remember that Aesculapius was famous for his unique method of healing the sick during sleep by making use of dreams to bring healing suggestions to bear on his patients. All this is a clear example of the use of the snake as an embodiment of the unconscious, that seed-bed of new and hitherto undreamed-of powers of healing. Thus the snake comes to be known as the symbol of re-birth, and this idea is supported by the belief in its immortality based on its annual habit of casting its skin.[2] Because of this idea of immortality, it comes to be considered as the symbol for the soul in general. Thus in Africa the dead reappear as snakes; in Greece the soul of the hero returns from the grave as a snake. To the Greeks, the serpent and the bird are soul animals[3] in different aspects; the serpent is the earth-soul, the bird the spiritual soul; and for this reason both are sacred to Athene.[4] For the Romans, the serpent is the incarnation of the Genius and Juno.[5] It is the earth-soul which gives man magic power.[6] In the Dionysian Sabazios mysteries of Asia Minor a golden serpent was passed through the garments of the initiant as a symbol of identification with the deity, which conferred redemption and immortality

[1] During a great plague in 293 B.C. the Romans sent an expedition to Epidauros in order to bring from there to Rome a serpent which was regarded as an incarnation of the god himself. (Chantepie de la Saussaye, Vol. II, p. 462.)

[2] Cf. the examples in Frazer, *Folklore in the Old Testament*, Macmillan, London, 1919, Vol. I, p. 50, 66ff., 75f.

[3] Chantepie de la Saussaye, Vol. II, p. 298.

[4] Ibid., p. 317.

[5] Ibid., p. 433. Genius and Juno were originally not specific deities, but personifications of the individual soul power of each human being, the Genius being the divine representative of the masculine generative power, and Juno that of the woman's function of conceiving and giving birth. (Ibid., p. 436.)

[6] Cf. for example the legend of Erechtheus and Cecrops (Preller, Vol. I, p. 198ff.). The Lithuanians have one and the same word for life and snake, namely "gyvata" (Chantepie de la Saussaye, Vol. II, p. 529).

on the soul.[1] These examples could be multiplied indefinitely, especially from Egyptian,[2] and above all from Indian mythology, in which the snake plays a prominent part. It is only necessary to mention the Kundalini serpent, which appears in Kundalini Yoga as the central power of the soul,[3] and also the symbol of the world-snake Shesha or Ananta, the animal of Vishnu/Krishna.[4]

Enough, however, has been said to illustrate the symbolical importance of the snake; it is the personification of the chthonic earthly unconscious, of the instinctual layer, with all its secret magic, mantic, and curative power, as well as its inherent dangers, which must be overcome. It is precisely this ambiguity which explains the veneration and also the fear inspired by the snake. As long as it retains the mastery, and its power in the depths of the human psyche has not been integrated, it is like a destructive poison, like the Flood overwhelming man's ego-consciousness. If he can subdue this force and integrate it into his consciousness, it will be transformed into a power for good, bestowing secret knowledge and the gift of spiritual rebirth.

Having thus explained the symbolical meaning of the three animals which appear in the dream, we can now tackle the actual interpretation of the dream itself.

As already mentioned, the first part of the dream (the boring party) corresponds to the everyday life of the dreamer; it represents the conscious level, where the I, the ego, stands in the centre of the field of consciousness.[5]

In moving to the adjoining room, he is leaving the psychic sphere in which he spends his social, and incidentally very bor-

---

[1]de Jong, *Antikes Mysterienwesen*, Brill, Leyden, 1909, p. 66; Preller, Vol. I, p. 701f.

[2]It is interesting that in Egypt it was customary to put a snake after the word for "goddess," and a falcon after the word for "god"—a significant psychological contribution to the understanding of the feminine and the masculine soul-power (and also to the conceptions of anima and animus). Adolf Erman, *Die Religion der Aegypter*, de Gruyter, Berlin, 1934, p. 45.

[3]Cf. Avalon, *The Serpent Power*, Ganesh, Madras, 1924.

[4]Cf. Zimmer, *Maja*, Stuttgart, 1936, pp. 44, 111 and elsewhere; Glasenapp, *Der Hinduismus*, Wolff, Munich, 1922, pp. 73, 229.

[5]Jung, *Psychological Types*, p. 540.

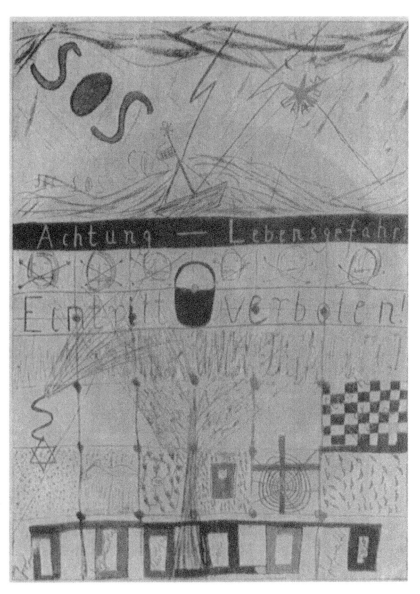

5.   Entrance Prohibited

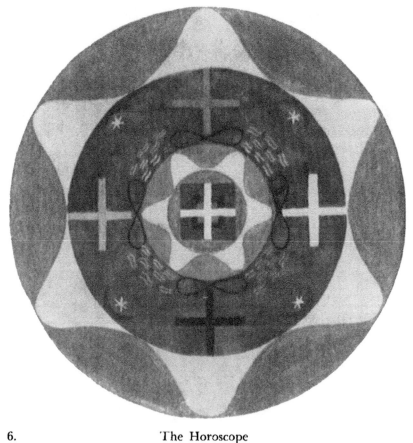

6.   The Horoscope

ing daily life. He enters a second room, in which he finds himself confronted with the, or put more accurately with "his," animals. In other words, in his dream he passes from the level of the ego and enters the world of the instincts. The symbolism of the animals, bear and wolf, will be most intimately connected with his particular psychological situation. The bear is a mother symbol; it represents, therefore, all those instincts which the dreamer has focused or projected on to his mother; the bear, in other words, is a personification of his infantile fixation on the mother-imago. As long as the bear remains *the* instinctual animal, it means that the dreamer's instincts are still undeveloped and primitive and entirely governed by an infantile desire to be pampered and spoiled. It is significant, however, that in this "room of the instincts," the dreamer is simultaneously confronted with the opposite of the bear, namely the wolf. It is interesting that the wolf too contains a slight allusion to the maternal animal (the motive of Romulus and Remus, though even here the wolf appears as the animal which looks after children exposed in the wilderness, so that there is a definite reference to the wild character of the wolf); but that the principal meaning, as all the other traits show, is the uncannily wild, fierce, predatory and voracious character of animal nature. That is, the dreamer is immediately faced with the contradictory character of the instincts, for his desire for his mother's care and protection meets with its very opposite, the wild ungovernable fury and all-consuming greed of his instincts. It is symptomatic of his condition that during this episode he reassures the bear, telling him to have no fear as he will take every precaution to prevent the wolf from doing him any harm. This portrays his attitude in a nutshell; the kind, indulgent mother corresponding to his infantile mother fixation, must at all costs be protected from any attack by the big, bad wolf, who, be it noted, is only a quarter its size. But the inexorable demands of life, the inherent law of psychological development, will not have it so; and in the end this law prevails. Although the wolf at first appears so small and "innocent," he proves in the sequel to be possessed of an uncanny superiority, and capable of rapidly assuming monstrous and terrible proportions, until in the end he is transformed into a being capable of encircling the world.

In order to understand this process, we must examine more closely the significant moment when the toy animals change into living creatures. To begin with, it is illuminating that the patient's instincts should masquerade as toy animals. It is characteristic of men of his type, namely intuitive intellectuals, that they aspire to live on a plane superior to the common necessities of life, including, of course, the basic demands of the instincts and desires. The patient's overpowering fear of his instincts and of the strength of his desires forced him during more than ten years to cling convulsively to an airy phantom, as by so doing he was enabled effectively to prevent, although at a terrible cost to himself, the realization of his instincts and emotional needs. This meant that, on the one hand, his instincts remained puerile and embryonic, only too easily satisfied with a toy world of make believe and phantasy (hence the toy animals) and on the other hand the repression of the true force of his instincts caused them to retaliate by reappearing in their most brutal and primitive form, as shown in the figure of the wolf. The gradual transformation of the animals into living creatures, which proceeds step by step with uncanny logic, reveals all their potential energy. The mere fact of his touching them sets in motion their hidden life; in other words he has only to penetrate to the instinctual level to find that, instead of having to deal with mere harmless, irresponsible phantasies, he is brought up sharp by the full blast of the unresolved problems threatening his very existence. It is, as it were, just "by chance," inadvertently, that he slips into this life and death contest with his own most fundamental problems.[1] Had

[1] The transition from the toy to the living animals is characteristic of the indirect approach which "nature" so often takes. It allures us by playing, but hidden behind its play is the seriousness of existence. This is the "way of the snake," which appears to take an indistinct direction, although it leads inevitably to the goal. While the direct way would often be too frightening, this indirect way, with its enticing, playful détours, nevertheless leads man finally to its goal—and that of the unconscious. This process can be seen in the situation of many analysands at the beginning of their analysis. They do not come because they feel the

these animals not first appeared as toys, he would never have been able to overcome his fear of them, and would certainly not have dared to touch them. The consequence of so doing comes as a nasty shock and an unpleasant surprise, but at the same time it is *the* prerequisite for that process of growth which alone will enable him to achieve full maturity. It is significant that the stupendous act of coming to life is concentrated in the wolf: the bear's rôle is very subsidiary; at any rate we hear practically nothing more about him. The only bit of information we get, and that is largely deduction, is that the bear too has been trans-

---

necessity of undertaking the task of coming to terms with the unconscious and finding an answer to the whole problem of their existence, but on account of some more or less superficial symptom. They believe that the symptom is the decisive problem; if they suspected what a critical and agonizing process of coming to terms with the problems of their life as a whole lay ahead of them, they would perhaps not have the courage to undertake it. The "indirect approach," however, leads them right into the depths of their decisive problem. Step by step they arrive, inadvertently as it were, at deep levels which would otherwise have remained inaccessible to them owing to their fear.

There is a strange Egyptian legend of the birth of the god Anubis which reflects this psychological situation in mythological terms. (I am indebted for the reference to this myth to the seminar on children's dreams which Prof. Jung held at the E.T.H., Zürich in 1936-7; cf. also Adolf Erman, *Die Religion der Aegypter*, pp. 72, 86.) According to this myth, the jackal-headed god of the underworld, Anubis, was begotten inadvertently by Osiris with Nephthys, the wife of Set. All four are brothers and sisters, being the children of the earth-god Keb and the sky-goddess Nut. Osiris, as the sun-god, is the bright masculine principle, and his adversary Set the dark one; similarly, Isis and Nephthys are respectively the bright and the dark feminine principle. One of the designations of Anubis is "the Opener of the Way"; that is, he is the guide through the underworld. It is notable that this guide through the underworld originates from the union of the bright masculine with the dark feminine principle, and that this happens "inadvertently." Psychologically, this means that access to the unconscious, with its perils and its mysteries, is only possible through the fertilization of the dark feminine side of a man (and vice versa in the case of a woman), that is through the acceptance of the anima, which contains the hazards of life. The conscious side, the "differentiated function," represented by Osiris, always tries to remain on the level of consciousness and to take a road which as it were by-passes fate (since fate is always dark and uncanny); but this means eliminating the unconscious possibilities. It is only "inadvertently," that is through a fate which lies outside conscious intention, that the conscious mind becomes involved with the depths of the unconscious—but if things go well, this leads to the birth of the "Opener of the Way." A man's real "fate" never comes to pass by means of the will and the differentiated side, but always through the side which is undifferentiated and near to nature, but for that very reason carries in it entirely new and unexpected potentialities. The conscious mind always wants to limit and define; new paths beyond these limits become available to man inadvertently, through the "Opener of the Way."

formed from a toy into a living animal ("I allow the wolf to claw
the bear's fur, telling him that he need not be afraid"); but the
dynamic force of the action is entirely focused on the development of the wolf.

A summary of the psychological interpretation of the dream
up to this point yields the following picture: On the plane of
everyday existence, the dreamer has stuck fast in a cul-de-sac,
since, owing to his mother-fixation and the resultant fears, he
is entirely cut off from the life-giving level of his instincts. His
unconscious leads him into the adjoining room, where he is confronted with his instincts. If we take the first room to represent
the level of the ego-consciousness, then it follows that the
"instinct-room" represents the level of the *personal unconscious*,
that is, the level of personal complexes and repressions. On this
level he is made to experience the conflict existing between the
infantile instincts centred on the mother-imago and the untamed
desires of the adult in all their natural strength. The covert suggestion contained in the pair of opposites mother-harlot is worth
noting, as this often represents the twin constellation under
which the primitive feeling of a man experiences the conflict between his infantile mother-fixation and the responsible acceptance of a really personal love relationship. His fear of facing the
problem casts an evil blight over any love relationship to a
woman other than his mother; and indeed, as long as the instincts
are uncontrolled and unintegrated—i.e. as long as they work as
"autonomous complexes"—they are a great danger. It is this
same fundamental fear of life which determines the gradual
awakening to life of the toy animals, a process which leads the
patient step by step, almost imperceptibly, to an examination
of his life's most crucial problem. A further stage in the solution
of his problem is indicated in the last part of the dream in which
the snake symbol forms the central motif.

From what has been said before, it follows that the snake expresses the ambiguity of nature, and is therefore peculiarly fitted
to symbolize the inherently contradictory character of psychic
factors. On the one hand, the snake is "the great dragon, that old

serpent, called the Devil, and Satan, which deceiveth the whole world";[1] on the other hand, it is the creature of salvation, the divine symbol, whom to accept and obey brings about the release and salvation of the soul.[2] Thus the snake expresses the ambivalence of earthly existence, for it is a constantly recurring question how far acceptance of this earthly life, of the "here and now," necessarily tarnishes the "heavenly radiance" of the "pure immortal soul." Nevertheless, the psychological fact remains that we are *also* of the earth, earthy, and that only by accepting this our earthliness can we develop into full-grown and integrated human beings. It is the failure to realize this difficult fact which prevents so many infantile people from ever achieving a really satisfactory and mature love relationship, because since the mother is the pure "unblemished" woman, every other woman seems a "temptress," from whose clutches he must flee to hide beneath the protective folds of the Madonna's sky-blue mantle. That is why "kissing the serpent" or "eating the serpent" forms the focal point of the mystery cult, since it expresses ceremonially the conquest of this fear,[3] a conquest which alone gives man the dominion over *this* world and thereby hope of the spiritual world beyond. Those for whom the snake is still a negative symbol remain subject to it; only when its positive meaning is realized can it be assimilated, and the world of the "here and now," of the desires and instincts, be fully integrated. This achievement also confers on the initiate the "wisdom of the serpent," and he is finally discharged from the womb of the

[1] *Revelation of St. John*, xii, 9.

[2] Cf. St. John iii, 14: "And as Moses lifted up the serpent in the wilderness, even so must the Son of Man be lifted up." For certain Gnostic sects—the Ophites —the serpent was Jesus. (Cf. Leisegang, *Gnosis*, p. 112: "Thus there was to be found here (in the Bible) in rich abundance all the material which made it possible to regard the serpent now as the Logos and the Saviour, now as the devil; to see in it the God who encircles the world (cf. the text of the dream) or as the Holy Spirit which enters into man and makes him a spiritual being.")

[3] Cf. Jung, *Psychology of the Unconscious*, p. 207. Cf. also Silberer, *Problems of Mysticism and Its Symbolism*, New York, 1917, p. 276: "The anxiety serpent is the 'guardian of the threshold' of the occultists; it is the treasure-guarding dragon of the myth. In mystic work the serpent must be overcome; we must settle with the conflict which is the serpent's soul."

mother-imago and assumes full maturity and a self-reliant, independent individuality. As soon as this soul-searching ordeal has been surmounted, the level of merely personal experience has already been left behind, and an insight has been gained into the realm of the eternal super-personal laws which govern life.

It is interesting in this connection to notice that the growth of the wolf to gigantic proportions and his transformation into the serpent take place "outside," indicating that the bounds of the particular personality have already been transcended. The room in which the patient finds his animals is still a part of his own personal psychology, it represents the instinctual level of the personal unconscious; still belonging to his own "dwelling-place." Beyond this, i.e. "outside," means that the limits of the particular personality have already been exceeded. The experience of the snake as the "adversary" belongs already to the level of the *collective unconscious,* of the "outside," that is to a level of the psyche existing beyond the range of merely personal experience. The dream shows quite clearly that the dreamer is not yet in the least capable of fully understanding and assimilating this very searching and far-reaching experience, but that, on the contrary, his infantile fears are still strong enough to give the experience a negative quality which effectually warns him off.

It is precisely at this stage that the *drawings* appear (cf. picture 10, page 160). Before discussing them I want to repeat a few technical remarks.[1] Analytical Psychology not infrequently makes use of drawings in its therapeutic work. They play an important part in the technique of *active imagination*. By active imagination we understand an intentional concentration on the processes taking place in the unconscious psychic hinterland; in other words it consists of a kind of "active passivity," enabling the patient, so to speak, to catch glimpses of his unconscious processes without interfering with them by the exercise of his conscious will. The attitude of mind necessary for this process cannot al-

[1] For a fuller description of the technique of "active imagination" cf. the preceding essay on the "Technique of Analytical Psychology."

ways be easily achieved, but not infrequently the desire for such a means of expression arises spontaneously out of the analytical situation. This is what happened in the case under discussion. A whole series of pictures came into being quite spontaneously, growing out of the first picture which the patient drew in response to my suggestion, namely that he should endeavour to make a drawing of the leit-motif of his dream. These drawings form a new and important development of the dream, so that one might really call them its continuation. In the dream the patient had touched a particularly crucial problem which clamoured for symbolical expression. The negative character of the dream expresses clearly his fear of facing the problems of his emotions and of his instinctual life. The fact, however, that he is now no longer willing to run away from his fear but is prepared to face and to overcome it, changes the whole situation. He has succeeded in realizing the meaning of his dream; thus he has won a new outlook and a higher level of consciousness, at which the positive and *progressive* aspects of the dream-symbols can become effective. It is through the process of active imagination that he approaches these positive contents; and they find expression in the symbolism of the drawings, in contradistinction to the dream. The value of such drawings lies precisely in the fact that these unconscious pictures possess a special symbolical power, for they come upon us with the full impact of a vision, not yet watered down by any rationalistic process. A pictorial symbolical expression, like every other symbol, possesses "magic" power; which explains, to quote but one instance, the important rôle played in many religions by sacred pictures and statues.

I do not propose in my discussion of these pictures to embark on an exhaustive survey of their far-reaching symbolism, but will confine myself to their direct and practical bearing on the patient's psychological problem.

The first picture (Fig. 1) is simply a representation of the motif already appearing in the dream, namely the giant snake encircling the world. If this were the only picture available, it would scarcely enable us to deduce anything more than what we already know from the contents of the dream itself. It does, however, in one important particular show an advance beyond the dream, namely that the snake is now invested with positive qualities as against its previously merely negative aspect. I refer to its crown of light rays, an attribute which reappears constantly throughout all the remaining series. This is important because it shows that the process of active imagination is penetrating to depths of the unconscious which are no longer subject to the dreamer's fear complex. In the dream the snake, coloured by the patient's fear of his instincts, appeared as the Adversary. Through his willingness, however, to face his fear, the symbols reveal their positive meaning, no longer influenced or falsified by the patient's personal complex. It is just this which gives the process of active imagination its potential value, namely that it penetrates behind the façade of personal fears and complexes and reveals the constructive and prospective potentialities contained in the experience. This is very important for the practical analysis of the dream, since it helps the patient to discover what complex is preventing him from possessing and making full use of his latent powers for good.

The next picture (Fig. 2) reveals that a process of differentiation is setting in, a process already latent in the first picture. The first picture represented the world and the serpent encircling it. The drawing reminds one of archaic cosmogonies in which two primeval forces create life out of themselves. The snake is the *demiurgos,* the creator of the world, who fertilizes matter, the maternal element. The second picture represents a further stage. Matter surrounded by the snake as demiurge begins to differentiate by contraction and splitting. The product of this process of fertilization and development is a new third element characterized by its blue colour as water.

This process of differentiation is carried a step further in the following picture (Fig. 3). In this a multitude of new worlds have been formed, each possessing its own little saviour snake, which is an exact replica of the original one. A comprehensive development and differentiation of the earth element has taken place. This picture forms the climax of the series. It is followed immediately by a very surprising anticlimax in the next picture (Fig. 4) which presents a spectacle of complete disintegration of the earth element. The worlds and their snakes have all disappeared, except for a few rudimentary fragments, faintly reminiscent of their former shape. The original snake has been reduced to a circle. The snake which was originally green is shading into blue; the earth is in process of dissolution; whereas blue, that is the water element which first appeared in the second picture, is now completely in the ascendant.

The fifth and last picture (Fig. 5) shows the process completed. The original snake, as well as all the later subsidiary snakes, have disappeared, so has the earth; all that remains is the blue element which seems however to have given birth to a tiny replica of itself.

What then is the psychological significance of this development? In the dream the feminine principle was first experienced by the dreamer as the mother (=bear); this purely infantile principle was partnered by the opposite principle, the harlot, personifying instinct and sexual desire. The snake in its ambivalent character represents the next stage; at first its negative aspect as the adversary is stressed, but later in the drawings, which represent the next step, its prospective and creative aspects are symbolized by the "saviour snake." The acceptance and integration of the unconscious layer indicate a decisive enlargement of consciousness, a new creative realization. The snake, originally a symbol inspiring fear, has thus become *nous*, wisdom, and creative power. Because of this newly won knowledge the undifferentiated matter becomes differentiated and fertile. This is shown in the drawings by the differentiation of the earth. Matter (=materia) is, as its name implies, maternal and feminine. The newly found knowledge and wisdom resulting from the acceptance of the instinctual level transforms the heavy unconsciously clinging maternal element into an individualized productive matrix for a new development, which will lead to the birth of a new element, water.

Taken as a whole, the pictures show two related and simultaneous processes; the one is the disintegration of the snake, the other the formation of water, which takes the place of the earth. The third picture, representing the individual earth spheres encircled by their own individual snakes, marks a definite turning-point, forming as it were the crisis of this line of development. The crisis in the picture corresponds exactly to a crisis in the psychological development. The encounter with the contents of the unconscious in all their power and autonomy carries with it the risk of being submerged and split up beneath its floodwaters, a danger which must be carefully kept in mind. In this sense the experience of becoming conscious of the contents of the collective unconscious resembles an artificially induced psychosis, and requires very careful handling on the part of the analyst, who at this stage of the analysis must maintain intact the patient's connection with reality. These pictures form a diagrammatic representation of the unconscious psychology of the patient, so that it is important that all the various worlds with their snakes should be confined within one vast serpent ring operating, as it were, as a magic protective circle against the danger of being split up. This protective circle is the "temenos,"[1] enshrining the august and holy place, the sacred grove, where the "numinous" event takes place. Because of the intensity and significance of this numinous process taking place within, the borders of the temenos must coincide with the magic circle. Not only must the "numinosum" inside be protected from the influx of outside influences, but the outside must also be guarded against a breaking through of the "numinosum"; for such a breakthrough would be tantamount to a psychosis.[2]

This point is of particular importance if we bear in mind the

[1]Cf. Jung, *The Integration of the Personality*, pp. 120 and 132; also the vision on p. 106, where a snake draws a circle about the dreamer.

[2]Cf. ibid., pp. 154 and 165.

fact that the patient is a schizophrenic borderline personality. The disruptive tendencies inherent in such a personality obviously demand special care. In the dream the disruptive tendencies are expressed by the figure of the wolf who changes into the giant snake. If this tendency were to get the upper hand, there would be a definite risk of the patient overstepping the danger line. The split in his personality can be defined as a split produced by the tension between the sphere of differentiated intellect and that of primitive feeling, between "Logos" and "Eros."[1] The task of the analysis is therefore to integrate within the patient's consciousness the disruptive tendencies which spring from primitive and still unconscious levels of feeling. This integration, however, can only be achieved if the patient can be brought to realize consciously the progressive side of these feeling contents, whereas so far he has only experienced them as a menace. This is exactly what happens in and through the drawings.

In this connection it is particularly important that the process of development should take place within the snake-ring, or magic circle. The third drawing shows clearly the danger of dissociation lurking within the patient's personality. Here the original tendency towards disruption, as symbolized by the snake (wolf) in the dream, is fully unfolded and exposed as shown by the propagation of the snakes. But they are held in check and kept within the bounds of the magic circle by the one saviour-snake, which encompasses and binds them together. Thus the third drawing expresses the instinctive effort to hold and weld together these disruptive tendencies, without, however, any longer placing an excessive strain on the intellect (with a corresponding repression of feeling), but control is achieved by means of the "snake-like wisdom" of the instinct and of Eros. The snake-ring of the third drawing is, so to speak, a symbolical representation of the alchemist's retort, of the "krater," where the process of synthesis takes place. This "alchemistic" process results in the formation of the new blue element, representing

[1] Cf. Jung, "Woman in Europe," in *Contributions to Analytical Psychology.*

the birth of individuality, or the identity of the personality, thus checking the danger of schizophrenic disruption and preparing the way for the assimilation of feeling. The new blue element is the real aim of the process of development which we have described, whereby a microcosm is differentiated out of a macrocosm; for whereas the macrocosm symbolizes the collective unconscious as matrix, the microcosm is the symbol of individuality.

It is interesting to note that a parallel type of symbolism is found in alchemy, which contained, alongside its chemical aspect, a philosophical concept of the birth and growth of the inner spiritual personality. Jung has dealt extensively with the symbolical aspect of alchemy, e.g. in his book on *Psychology and Religion,* from which most of the following parallels are taken. One of the fundamental ideas of alchemy is the redistillation from its chaotic concomitants of the divine spirit hidden in matter.[1] To accomplish this process the chemical element Mercury is absolutely indispensable, and this element is called by the alchemists "Mercurius animatus," "serpent" or "dragon."[2] The Mercurius of the alchemists "was understood to be a Hermes psychopompos, showing the way to the Paradise."[3] Thus we meet here again the serpent with the help of which the divine spirit is to be redistilled from undifferentiated matter. This extract, the famous tinctura, is also represented as a blue miraculous fluid which one of the most famous alchemists called also *"le ciel humain."*[4] This miraculous blue liquid, the tinctura, was also given the symbol of the circle. To the alchemists the circle is the symbol of the macrocosm and of divine perfection;[5] and it is interesting to note that the point, the microcosm, is spoken of as the "creative point in matter" and as "the soul spark."[6] Expressed psychologically, the birth of the blue microcosm out of the macrocosm in our drawings points to the birth of the patient's individuality out of the matrix of the collective unconscious,

[1] Jung, *Psychology and Religion,* New Haven, 1938, p. 109.
[2] Silberer, *Problems of Mysticism and Its Symbolism,* p. 155. Cf. also p. 115.
[3] Jung, *Psychology and Religion,* p. 128.
[4] Ibid., p. 109.
[5] Ibid., pp. 66, 128.
[6] Ibid., p. 124.

which has been achieved in the development just described.

To sum up, the main theme of the drawings is that of the creation of a new world. Through the encounter with the wolf which then turns into the snake, his infantile dream world is destroyed. The realization that he has to leave his child's paradise, and the conquest of the fear of this step, reveals the snake as demiurgos, and his own psychic world is created. Instead of the mother who has so far been to him the sole source of creation, the snake as demiurgos reveals his own inner creativeness, and thus he need no longer be "bored." Each human being is, as it were, the small demiurge of a small psychic world of his own, and thus the patient becomes an equal to other people. The snake is *nous*, wisdom and creative realization, and through a deeper and more adequate realization of his own nature in particular and human nature in general—i.e. of the inner psychic laws—he creates his own world, and with it his own individuality. So far the microcosm of his individuality is still undifferentiated (cf. Fig. 5), as he has still to plunge into the problems of life which he has so far evaded; but at least he is now willing and prepared to come to grips with them. The change from the original green of the drawings to the ultimate blue finally symbolizes the creation of a new, living spirit through the inclusion of nature (=snake) and earth into his personality.

Translated into terms of practical life, this means that the patient no longer projects his emotional difficulties on to some outside person, that is, he ceases to hang them round the neck of his imaginary lady-love, but on the contrary faces up to them as contents of his own psychological make-up with which he is required to deal. Even if this result appears banal compared with the far-reaching symbolism of dream and drawings, it is of decisive importance to the patient. For it shows the way to the achievement of personal integration and to the healing of the split between Logos and Eros which had hitherto kept the whole of the emotional side of his life suppressed and therefore rudimentary. It was significant that a few weeks after this dream the patient made the acquaintance of a young girl with whom he was soon on very happy terms of close friendship. Evidently his feelings and emotions, which had hitherto been completely chained to the projected figure of his imaginary love, were now free and capable of fulfilling their purpose in real life. To put it in another way, the power of the mother-imago and of his infantile protective system had been broken down. Such an achievement is necessarily accompanied by growth in spiritual maturity—issuing in the birth of an independent and self-reliant individuality. This process is symbolized in the last drawing where the blue macrocosm and microcosm are shown as the end result of the present development.

From the point of view of technique I should like to stress the fact that at that stage of the analysis I did not discuss with the patient the symbolism of the drawings in detail, but only gave him a rough idea of their meaning.[1] In particular I pointed out to him the positive significance of the snake and of the birth of a new principle. The realization of these two facts, closely related as they were to his feeling problem, was just what he needed at that time, and was therefore quite sufficient to set in motion the process of psychological development.

It is evident that the drawings corresponded to a profound and very definite psychological need of the patient. In them he experiences the birth of a world of his own, instead of the obsolete infantile one. They help to create a potential for his psychic energy, his libido; they are, as it were, principles of direction, they form a chart whereby to steer his future course. The new idea they contain, namely that the acceptance of the instincts and emotions means the deliverance of his own individuality, gives him the courage to venture upon the dangerous step onto the other unknown shore. That this was indeed his response in real life is shown by his actual achievement of a successful love relationship. Speaking generally, such symbols help to build a bridge between present consciousness and the future goal; they are a diagram of the entelechy of the individual personality.

[1]In order to dispel a possible objection it may be important to point out that at the time when the patient produced the drawings, Jung had not yet published any of his books on the psychological symbolism of alchemy. Neither the patient nor myself were acquainted at the time with this aspect of his symbols.

Such symbols however are not merely principles of direction, but they are at the same time an actual source of energy. The symbolism of the pictures was not drawn from the patient's personal experiences, but issued from the storehouse of the collective unconscious which disposes of quite other experiences and means than are open to merely personal knowledge. It is for this very reason that the technique of active imagination is so valuable in our work, for it offers our patients access to the symbols of the collective unconscious. The individual himself is only aware of his own dire need and the danger into which his problem has precipitated him and from which, owing to his fear and to his limited personal experience, he can see no way of escape. The symbolism of the collective unconscious, however, because of its infinitely greater experience of such critical situations, reveals it to him in its true colours as a typical crisis of growth of human consciousness from which the fruit will develop in due season. The admission and recognition of the true meaning of the situation frees psychic energies which were hitherto beyond reach and therefore incapable of being utilized. With their help the individual no longer feels isolated and adrift on a limitless ocean, but realizes himself as an individual instance of the typical story of human crises and decisions.

NOTE

The colours of the original drawings are as follows:

In Fig. 1 the snake has a dark green colour, with a yellow crown of rays, and a red tongue. The earth has a brown-yellowish colour.

In Fig. 2 the colour of snake and earth has remained the same; the space between snake and the three globes is blue.

The colours in Fig. 3 correspond to those of the two previous ones; green snakes with yellow crowns and red tongues, brown-yellowish globes, and blue in between.

In Fig. 4 the green snake has turned into a blue-green ring, the fragments have a yellowish green colour, whereas the original blue has remained.

The last drawing shows a plain blue colouring.

IV

THE EGO AND THE CYCLE
OF LIFE

With the drawing of this Love and the voice of this Calling
We shall not cease from exploration
And the end of all our exploring
Will be to arrive where we started
And know the place for the first time. . . .
T. S. Eliot, Little Gidding. (1942).

ACCORDING to an old cabalistic legend describing the
"Formation of the Child,"[1] God ordains that at the moment of
creation the seed of the future human being shall be brought
before Him, whereupon He decides what its soul shall become:
man or woman, sage or simpleton, rich or poor. Only one thing
He leaves undecided, namely whether he shall be righteous or
unrighteous, for, as it is written, "All things are in the hand of
the Lord, except the fear of the Lord." The soul, however,
pleads with God not to be sent from the life beyond this world.
But God makes answer: "The world to which I send thee, is
better than the world in which thou wast; and when I formed
thee, I formed thee for this earthly fate." Thereupon God
orders the angel in charge of the souls living in the Beyond to
initiate this soul into all the mysteries of that other world,
through Paradise and Hell. In such manner the soul experiences
all the secrets of the Beyond. At the moment of birth, however,
when the soul comes to earth, the angel extinguishes the light of
knowledge burning above it, and the soul, enclosed in its earthly

---

[1]Cf. Angelo S. Rappoport, *The Folklore of the Jews,* Soncino, London, 1937, p. 92.

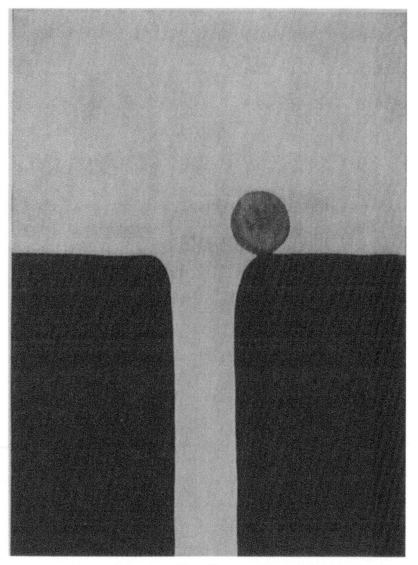

7. The Abyss

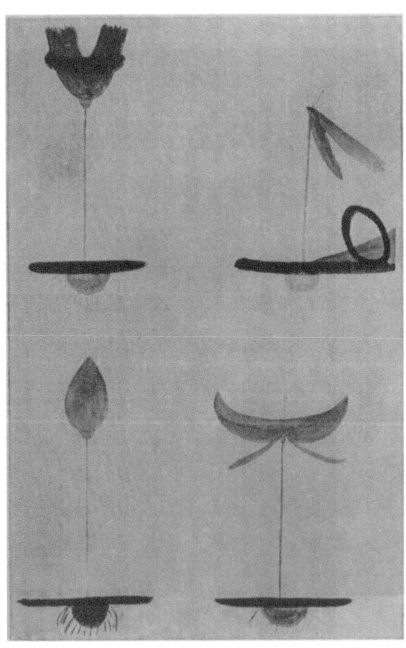

8.   The Two Flowers

envelope, enters this world, having forgotten its lofty wisdom, but always seeking to regain it.

What is the psychological meaning of this profound myth regarding the fate of the soul? According to the legend, God ordains the future development of the seed, but with one curious and extremely significant limitation. He does not ordain whether the seed shall develop into the soul of a righteous or of an unrighteous man, for "all things are in the hand of the Lord, except the fear of the Lord." This means that a certain fate and a certain way are laid down for each man, but whether he fulfils this fate and goes his appointed way or not remains in his own power. For the "fear of the Lord," the willing acceptance of His divinely appointed purpose, that is: the element of ethical choice, remains within the individual's power. The goal is fixed, but the way of approach and its achievement are left to each individual. Truly a profound answer to the eternal problem of free will! In the dialogue with God, the soul, fearing to lose her purity by contact with the transitoriness of earthly existence, protests against having to descend into this world. But God rebukes her. The world she is about to enter is better than the former one, seeing that this is the world for which the soul was created. In other words, the whole meaning of the existence of every soul lies precisely in the fact that she can only achieve her ultimate meaning in and through the realities of this actual earthly world. The real purpose and object of the soul does not consist in the achievement of a purely sinless state in an ideal world, but rather in the willing acceptance of the responsibilities of this concrete world and the constantly recurring obligation of choice which they entail. That is why, although before birth the soul is acquainted with all the secrets of the Beyond, the moment she enters this world she must forget all that knowledge in order to discover it afresh in and through her experience in this life and so make it her very own.

What however does the world of the Beyond, from which the soul originates, mean in psychological language? The "Beyond" is the repository of the ultimate secrets of heaven and hell, of light and darkness, above and below, positive and negative—in other words it is the world of the collective unconscious from which we all originate. It is not without reason that the fairy tale of the stork who fetches children out of the deep lake is so persistent—for it is only another presentation of the same psychic experience, namely that we all spring from these great waters. For it is not true, as has been stated by a mechanistic and one-sidedly rationalistic psychology, that man is born a *tabula rasa* and a blank page. On the contrary, he conceals within the depths of his being experiences dating from archaic times, and traces of countless actions and reactions going far beyond the bounds of personal existence, just as certain individual possibilities are already foreshadowed within him which point to a time reaching far into the future. It is of the very essence of the child that it still lives in the mysterious world of mythical images and magical relatedness; indeed it is immersed in the world of the images of the collective unconscious, of the mythological past of mankind which is as yet undimmed by the concrete realities of the present. The great collective images of the past are still so near and powerful in the case of a child that his first task is to free himself from the fascination of their super-personal power, and in conflict with these forces he must forge his own small personality, thus extricating and developing his still very fragmentary individual ego.

If we wish to understand the psychology of a small child we must therefore approach it from the angle of a world of myth and magic, in which psychologically speaking its life has not yet achieved any individual name but exists in a purely anonymous state. Everyone who has ever had any dealings with children has met with countless instances which can only be explained in relation to this anonymous mythical and magical sphere. For example, nearly all children practise certain peculiar ceremonies, especially at bedtime, for the transition from waking to sleeping is of particular importance, representing as it does the mysterious moment of transition from light to darkness. These ceremonies may consist in some ritualistic way of bidding good night, or carefully shaking hands with the dolls, or similar procedures. These puerilities, which can be so easily disregarded, are, properly considered, survivals of magic apotropaic, that is protective ceremonies, customary in primitive races. Just because a child has an instinctive knowledge of the minuteness of its own small ego as opposed to the primeval force of the collective powers, it seeks by means of such ceremonies before going to sleep to ensure that its tiny ego will not be completely reabsorbed into the lap of the great primeval night. We adults forget too easily what a terrifying experience it is to a child to see the light disappear—indeed, is there any guarantee that light and life will re-appear again? But at least, if things are to-night as they have been yesterday and the day before, there is some hope that they will be the same again tomorrow. Jung has given an account of an interesting ritual of the Pueblo Indians of Mexico among whom he lived for some time. They regard themselves as children of the sun, and it is their sacred duty to make the sun rise every morning by certain ritual performances. If they were to abandon this ritual the sun would, after some time, cease to rise again. This is a clear projection and concretization of psychological danger; without certain ritual observances the light of consciousness would be lost. In the same way the ceremonies of children represent magic spells against the great forces of darkness so that the tiny light of the child's individuality may not be extinguished.

An interesting commentary on this is furnished by the remark of a five-year-old child who, on being questioned about its dreams, answered: "The dream is not in my head, but I am in the dream."[1] For children are actually enclosed within their dreams, that is within the all-enveloping power of the great psychic primeval night. That is why children so easily confuse reality and phantasy, the dividing line between the two being at first almost non-existent. I remember a child of six which was overjoyed one morning because it had dreamed in the night

[1] Jean Piaget, *La pensée symbolique et la pensée de l'enfant.* In: Arch. de psychol. 1923, XVIII. ("Moi je suis dans le rêve, le rêve n'est pas dans ma tête.")

that it had been given a very beautiful doll with which it had been playing; and this feeling of happiness remained even after waking because the dream present was for the child an absolutely real and concrete fact. Another example, to which one could easily find parallels, is that of a boy of four-and-a-half, who, on seeing a picture of a soldier shooting another one dead, promptly took his toy gun and shot the murderer dead, subsequently heaving a sigh of relief,[1] because the murder, from his point of view, had thus not only been avenged in the world of phantasy but also in actual fact. A well-known example in literature of the magic rites practised by youths can be found in Rousseau's *Confessions,* where he relates how in his boyhood, he made use of an oracle. He used to aim a stone at a tree. If he hit the tree he took this as a good omen, if he missed, it was a bad sign. (The tree, by the way, had to be of a reasonable size in order not to make his task too difficult!) Indeed, who among us grown-up people is quite emancipated from all magic practices, in spite of labelling them as mere "superstitions," practices such as making a secret wish at the sight of a falling star or not treading on the cracks between the paving stones?

This magical thinking is typical of a certain level of life which is rooted not so much in the personal ego but in the impersonal layer of the collective unconscious. An excellent outcrop of this layer can be observed in the artistic efforts of children. There is, for example, the drawing of a five-year-old girl (cf. picture 18, page 224). This is an entirely spontaneous expression of feeling without any definite subject. But its contemplation creates quite unmistakably the impression of a mythical landscape or of a picture which might have come from the world of the Arabian Nights. It is remarkable what a strong emotional effect may be produced by such a completely naïve picture by a child. But this is understandable because it is nothing more nor less than the expression of the child's inner landscape, if one may use that phrase; it is in fact a statement which expresses the colour and

[1] E. and G. Scupin, *Bubi im* 4–6 *Lebensjahr,* Leipzig, 1910, p. 126.

tension of the child's mythical interior world in which the greater part of its life is lived. This spontaneity and intensity, however, is only possible because of the enormous preponderance and vitality of this mythical world compared to the world of the ego-consciousness.

In the case of the ordinary adult the barrier erected by the ego-consciousness against the world of collective images is so high that, generally speaking, it can only be surmounted with difficulty. This also explains the peculiar psychology of the artist. Starting from the world of his ego-consciousness and with its help he is able to extend his adventures into the world of myth and magic. Like Ulysses, safely bound to the mast of reality, he is yet able to listen to the siren voices and incorporate their music in his songs. For this reason poets have in all ages been reckoned among the wise men of a people. They are the "seers," that is, they see the great super-personal interrelations in the universe. Whereas a child may be said to lead a unipolar life, a life functioning mainly in the layer of the collective unconscious, the artist's life is bipolar; in the full possession of his own ego he descends into the underworld of the collective images, and through the medium of his own individual personality he offers his awestruck audience treasure-trove from the deep. That is why an artist lives in perpetual danger of being submerged beneath the overwhelming waves of the great collective images, and it is well known how only too often the powers of this magic world enslave and overpower and finally engulf him.

In this collective world of the artist and the child, magicians and fairies are not characters in a fairy tale but ordinary earthly inhabitants. Characteristic examples of such artistic creation are two figures by a boy of five-and-a-half years, which he drew, cut out and painted entirely on his own initiative (cf. picture 11, page 161). The first consists of a strange daimonic figure, having a peculiar mythical headdress, consisting of a crown with one horn on each side, a figure which reminds one very forcibly of a primitive magician's dance mask, or the full warpaint of a medicine man. The second picture, drawn by the same boy, depicts a similar figure, a kind of demon, with a long tail, which may be also interpreted as an unconscious phallic symbol. In this case the headdress is even more elaborate, with its two

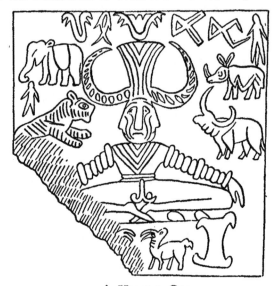

9. A HORNED GOD.
Reproduced from Margaret A. Murray: *The God of the Witches.*

enormous horns and a centre part which, as in the first figure appears to carry a peculiar mythical symbol at the apex. It is scarcely possible to imagine a better and more vivid representation of a magician or an animal-god.

The close parallelism between the child's mind and the images of the collective unconscious can be impressively illustrated by comparing these pictures with a picture dating from the Bronze Age. It is a representation from Mohenjo-Daro of the Indian god Prajapati,[1] "the Lord of all creatures," who personifies the creative powers of nature. The two demons of the child can easily be taken to represent his own instinctual creative

[1]From Margaret Alice Murray, *The God of the Witches*, Sampson Low, London (no year), Plate III.

energies. Especially striking is the amazing similarity in the headdress with the horns on either side, and the central column which in each case is crowned by another two-winged symbol. It is a clear indication of how strongly the phantasy of children is determined by the images of the collective unconscious.

If we sum up the main points we get the following picture of the child's psychological growth. Its development starts from a condition of complete participation in, and undifferentiation from, the inner and outer world in which it lives; it then proceeds by way of the development of its ego, and the separation of its personality from its anonymous identity with all existing facts. That is why the word "I" only enters the consciousness of the child comparatively late, towards the end of the third year of life; a sign that it is only then that the first appreciable and conscious traces of an ego-personality as opposed to the collective psyche appear.

It is an interesting parallel that primitive languages frequently have no expression for the ego. Thus "in the original Semitic language there exists no expression for the 'Ego.' The original Semite does not say 'I kill,' but: 'Here killing.' Only gradually there developed what we mean by saying 'I kill.' If the Maori speaks in the first person, he does not necessarily speak of himself but of his group, with which he naturally identifies himself. He says 'I' have done this or that and means thereby 'My tribe has done it.' 'My' soil means the land of the tribe."[1] This is, as with the child, a sign of the as yet fragmentary development of an ego-consciousness. This fact has been remarked upon by anthropologists with regard to practically every primitive civilization. Thus, to give only one example out of many, it has been said of the Kaffirs: "They are but dimly conscious of large tracts of their own individuality, which lie below the level of full consciousness. . . . The subliminal self is enormously greater than that portion of it which rises to full self-consciousness."[2]

[1] Hans Kelsen, *Society and Nature,* Kegan Paul, London, 1946, p. 11.
[2] Dudley Kidd, *The Essential Kaffir,* 1904; quoted from Hans Kelsen, l.c., p. 6.

But the attainment of a more and more comprehensive ego-consciousness indicates the direction in which the development of mankind in general and of the child and the adolescent in particular proceeds. Emancipation from the tremendous power of the collective images is an extraordinarily difficult process bristling with conflicts. In the case of primitives such attempts are extremely half-hearted, and are always accompanied by sacrificial offerings designed to placate the primeval forces.[1] Even in our own day, too many of us give up the attempt half-way or at the first obstacle. How seductive and enchanting is the prospect of remaining sheltered in this magic world—how cold and cruel appear the hard, sharp contours of the conscious ego in comparison. The infinite difficulties attendant on this emancipation are reflected in such myths as that of the First Fall, for the task of separation from "Paradise," which is, psychologically speaking, the state before differentiated consciousness, seems so enormous that it is felt to be sacrilege and sin.

The decisive break away from the state of identification with the world of collective psychic contents and with it the step into the world of the individual ego occurs only at puberty. The aggressiveness and self-assertiveness of adolescence are only the outward manifestation of this inner conflict, and the degree of revolt and aggressiveness reflect the strength of the conflict. It is interesting to note that primitive races only recognize puberty in a purely physical sense. The lengthy and painful process of psychic puberty during which the personality bursts through its previous chrysalis stage is as unknown to primitive races as is our conception of individual personality.[2] The initiation rites of adolescents serve therefore not so much to initiate the youth into the life of a fully developed individual as into

[1]"Any fresh form of activity, any new work undertaken for the first time, entails some magic peril on the doer, and it is therefore essential to combat it beforehand, by a preparation which is equally magic in its nature." (L. Lévy-Bruhl, *Primitives and the Supernatural*, Allen and Unwin, London, 1936, pp. 363f.)

[2]Cf. Margaret Mead, *Coming of Age in Samoa* (Penguin Books, Vol. A. 127), particularly Chapters IX and XIII.

a new level of collective life, that is, the social and religious activities of the tribe. "The main significance of initiation rituals, common among primitive peoples, is to bring the boys into rapport with the spirits of the ancestors, who guarantee the social order, and to induce initiated man, by ceremonies which produce fear and awe of the superhuman authorities, to obey the tribal customs."[1]

An excellent illustration of this struggle to achieve individuality is provided by the drawing of a boy of eleven, that is in the stage preceding puberty (cf. picture 12, page 168). The picture shows an enormous tree with a tremendously developed network of roots, the tree itself growing up between two monstrous dragons. A tiny little man with a knapsack above his head sits in the crown of the tree, obviously a hunter on the look-out, since a kind of spear is directed at one of the monsters. The meaning of the picture is this: The man stands for the specifically human element, that is the ego-consciousness. The dragons represent forces of the collective unconscious which must be overcome. It will easily be understood that they portray the psychic images of the parents, the all-powerful figures of the parental archetypes. For during childhood it is above all these archetypes which, as representatives of the collective unconscious, form the opposite pole to the individual ego; which also explains why the strength of the parental influence so greatly exceeds the actual personality of the parents. An interesting feature of the drawing is the fact that the dragon on the left is characterized by a moustache indicating the male, and therefore representing the father-archetype; the dragon on the right would therefore represent the maternal archetype. It is against this maternal archetype, the female dragon, that the spear is aimed, indicating that, for the time being, the first task confronting the boy is to free himself from his mother. The tree, on the other hand, represents the natural process of growth, the "way of life," a tree whose immense reptilian roots are firmly anchored in the primeval depths of the creating and nourishing earth, thus rendering it capable

[1]Kelsen, *Society and Nature*, p. 22. Cf. also p. 293.

of supporting the midget personality and saving it from the rapacious monsters which typify the impersonal collective images. For the unconscious has a double aspect: the productive and constructive on the one hand and the destructive and consuming on the other. As the dragons at this particular juncture of life represent the destructive aspect of psychic nature, so does the tree stand for a symbol of life with its unceasing and instinctive growth.

Indeed, the whole of life is a process of adaptation to certain *a priori* facts. We are born, but the realities of the outer world of facts surrounding us, as also the reality of the inner world—that is the world of the collective unconscious and of the archetypes—are pre-existent realities, eternally and all-powerfully present. Every individual is born anew into this world, with the inexplicable possession of a minute germ of ego-personality, the real X, or unknown factor in life, which must not only adapt itself to these inner and outer realities, but absorb them and relive them individually. Without this ego which has to experience and recreate the inner and outer realities, the whole of the world, psychologically speaking, would be non-existent. If the individual is able so to recreate the world within his own consciousness, then the totality of the universe has been enriched by the existence of his infinitesimal ego, and the world of the archetypes has been modified, be it ever so slightly. If he fails in this attempt, then the life of one individual human being has passed like a bubble rising from the primeval swamp and bursting into nothingness. Life in itself is nature, and nature has no conscious history. It is consciousness which creates time, and thereby creates history. It is of great significance that primitive races have no history in our sense of the word; for them, the life of the individual, just as the life of the tribe, waxes and wanes like the seasons and passes on without any history.[1] For without consciousness there is no time, and thus children as well as

[1] Cf. L. Lévy-Bruhl; *Primitive Mentality*, Allen and Unwin, London, 1923; pp. 89ff.; p. 384. Cf. also Ch. Letourneau, *La Psychologie ethnique* (1901) p. 40. "For the child there is scarcely a past and a future. Like the savage, it lives almost exclusively in the present moment" (quoted from Kelsen, l.c., p. 270).

primitives have only a weak sense of chronological order. It is only consciousness, personified by the individual ego, which introduces a new element. The processes of nature are in an endless circle. It is only the conscious ego which makes it possible to step outside this circle, and by contemplating it from outside, so to speak, to recreate it anew. Such is the enormous achievement of human consciousness. This is the stupendous act by which man separates himself from the purely natural web of circumstance and sets himself up as the opposite pole to nature, the promethean struggle which, because of its breathtaking onslaught on the purely natural order of things, is for ever calling down upon itself the wrath of the gods. Yet it is man's inescapable destiny to be for ever attempting this, since it is only through consciousness that man can attain to full humanity, and without consciousness he remains blind nature.

It is in the nature of man to possess in his inherent structure a tendency to individuation, a characteristic which we must accept although we cannot explain it scientifically, and this tendency works itself out in and through the objective facts of the outer and inner reality. Speaking psychologically, the consciousness of man is for ever recreating the world afresh, but conversely and simultaneously, it is being re-shaped by the actual facts of the world. The relationship between nature and ego, between the collective unconscious and the individual consciousness, is that of action and reaction, and it is precisely this mutual relationship which constitutes the reality of the human world.

This relationship of man and nature, of subject and object, is best expressed in the actual words "subject" and "object"; "*objectum*" means literally that which is in opposition, or facing you; "*subjectum*" that which is subjacent, subordinate, or at the mercy of the object. But the object can only attain life through the subject. The task of the first half of life therefore consists in establishing this subject so firmly that it is capable of acting as equal and opposite pole and as receptive agent to the *objectum*. But it is just because the *objectum* by its very nature is, at first, so overwhelmingly the stronger element in this partnership, that this task is so tremendously difficult. The *objectum* is dowered with the whole force of nature, and we are never allowed to forget that, from the point of view of nature, the fact of our ego-personality is an entirely superfluous, nay even harmful intrusion. For nature apparently has only one aim, that of self-propagation, or the purely biological conservation of life. From this point of view, our individuality appears a completely unnecessary luxury, nay more, an actual threat to these purely biological aims. That is why blind nature always seems to want contemptuously to snuff out our small luxury egos. Nevertheless, in spite of this disproportion in size, the urge towards individuation stands on a footing of equality with its opposite pole, pure nature, and the whole problem consists in resolving the thesis of pure nature and its antithesis of the opposing ego into the synthesis of *conscious* nature.

The tremendous tension which exists between a purely natural condition and that of ego-consciousness explains why it is so extraordinarily difficult for an individual to free himself from the psychic powers of the collective unconscious, and why this attempt so often fails. Thus a little girl of three-and-a-half asked her mother to put a great stone on her head because she did not want to die. She was asked how the stone would prevent it, and answered with perfect childish logic: "Because I shall not grow tall if you put a stone on my head; and people who grow tall get old and then die."[1] That is an example of the enormous retrograde attraction exercised by the state of primeval nature. Another similar example was related to me by a man in the middle thirties, who came to me suffering from a strong mother-fixation, and who was altogether very markedly identified with his family. He told me that as a small child he often dared not breathe deeply in case he should use up his breath prematurely, so that there would not be enough left over for the remainder of his life. Both cases are tragic examples of the fact that even in earliest childhood the fear of the next step or of the need for making future decisions may be so

[1] J. Sully, *Studies of Childhood*, London, 1895, p. 121.

marked that all possible expedients'are attempted in order to remain in the present, a present, alas, so fleeting that out of sheer longing for paradise the whole of this life is missed. This is the fear of losing the protective mantle cast by the primeval condition of identification with the collective unconscious, the fear in fact of becoming an individual and thereby assuming full human responsibility.

It is this same fear of the new and the unknown which makes primitive people so unbelievably conservative in their rites and customs. Every innovation necessitates a new adaptation, and the consequences might be too dangerous. A new fact does not arouse the curiosity of the primitive man but his fear.[1] Without his old customs primitive man finds himself lost in a whirlpool of bewildering facts. An intelligent Eskimo shaman said to Rasmussen: "Therefore it is that our fathers have inherited from their fathers all the old rules of life which are based on the experience and wisdom of generations. We do not know how, we cannot say why, but we keep those rules in order that we may live untroubled. And so ignorant are we in spite of all our shamans, that we fear everything unfamiliar. . . . Therefore we have our customs."[2]

To hold fast to every minute seems to give us a certain illusory feeling of protection, but at the cost of severe anxieties of another kind, for the tree of life grows inexorably upwards. The wheel rolls on, and if we remain stationary it rolls over us. He who tries to escape life, that is the development of his own individual personality, falls a victim to life. Only he who accepts life with all its complications and conflicts attains to full living consciousness, enabling him to find a new life-centre beyond the reach of present entanglements. Only by a full experience of life can we become conscious, and the tragedy of the situation lies precisely in the fact that it is only by separating

[1]Cf. Kelsen, l.c., p. 2.

[2]Rasmussen, *Intellectual Culture of the Iglulik Eskimos* (quoted from Kelsen, l.c., p. 22).—Numerous examples of this well-known hostility of primitives to every change or innovation—the so-called "misoneism"—can be found in Lévy-Bruhl's books; cf. *Primitives and the Supernatural* or *Primitive Mentality.*

ourselves from the collective matrix that we become capable of experience. As long as we remain identified with any fact of life we have not experienced it. The requirement of all knowledge and experience involves a separation of our ego from that which has always been, that is from the collective images, the archetypes. He who runs away from his experiences and refuses to make this act of separation, renders himself powerless against the dark forces of the underworld; he who will not look them straight in the eye is attacked by them from behind, and instead of integrating them he is overwhelmed by the dark shadow world of psychic nature.

The following dream may serve as a brief illustration of this. It was related to me some months after the beginning of the analysis by the same patient who as a child was afraid of breathing too deeply.

"I am in a field and am hacking up the earth with a pointed pickaxe. My two children are sitting beside me. Suddenly I see my parents who come to visit me, whereupon I experience an irresistible impulse to attack my children with the pickaxe."

This shows that the patient has already managed to emancipate himself to some extent from his family, and has gained a certain degree of individuation—for he is cultivating his own field with his "children" by his side. (In actual fact he was neither married nor had he children.) But the power of the parental imagines is still so overwhelming that their appearance causes him to transform the tool which he had hitherto been using productively into a deadly weapon against his "children," who in this case represent his own future development. In actual life, the patient had to pay for this tendency of his to sacrifice again and again the germ of his own personality to the dark powers of his ancestors, by terrible fears and obsessions.

As a pendant, the following dream of a young woman in the middle twenties is interesting. She had reached a critical point in her struggle to adapt herself to life and to accept her personal task and individual development. In this critical situation she dreamed:

"Snow-landscape. In front of me there is an ice-berg, concealing a man who wishes to work his way through the iceberg to me. I call to him ironically: 'You will never be able to do that, no one has yet accomplished it.' The man goes on working. Great pieces of ice fly out on all sides. I begin to get anxious about the man and am afraid that his strength will give out and that he will freeze to death. The ice-berg is transparent. I am anxiously trying to dig an opening into the iceberg with my hands. Now we are only a little way apart. I stretch out my hands to the man, saying: 'You must be frozen, take my hands, they are warm.' I draw him with my hands towards me . . . we kiss each other."

In a wonderful picture this dream shows how life, personified in the man, her natural opposite, approaches the woman whose neurotic fear of life is so great that she cannot believe that life will really reach her or she reach life. By her ironic cry she attempts to deny the call of life, but seized and transformed by its irresistible energy she decides in time to accept life and to meet it in a spirit of joyful co-operation. Thus the seemingly impossible has become the possible.

This is the direction in which every human being must necessarily proceed as he grows out of the identification of childhood towards the acceptance of the social and concrete responsibilities of adult life. Emancipation from father or mother means assuming the duties of a father or a mother oneself, whether this takes the form of founding a family, or exercising a profession, in short becoming a responsible member of society and accepting fully the world of external reality. Every stage of life has its specific duty, and he who does not fulfil these specific duties, that is who does not live through that particular phase, has failed to experience one aspect of life, and the price of this refusal is either stultification and numbness or a neurosis. The life process marches logically and irresistibly onwards, and woe betide him who seeks to evade its demands.

The child is born into the world without a proper ego, and the phase of childhood up to the age of puberty, that is roughly speaking the first decade of life, corresponds to the slow unfolding of the latent powers of the ego, and the gradual shelling out of the delicate little germ of individuality from the various layers of identifications and magic participations. The phase of puberty, that is roughly the second decade, involves severing the psychic umbilical cord connecting the growing individuality with the psychic womb of the family. In the next phase, that of the young man and the young woman, or the third decade, the ego becomes more coherent and self-reliant, and he or she, by coming to grips with the realities of life, attain their individuality. The fourth decade means the assimilation of the world, and the final achievement of its psychic conquest through the fulfilment of all its legitimate demands. This last phase involves the complete adaptation of man as a social being, and simultaneously the fulfilment of the main task of personality which is the achievement of a completely integrated ego-consciousness.

In the case of the average normal individual this task is usually accomplished by the fourth decade. In the ordinary way, a man has usually laid the ground-plan of his position in society by the end of the thirties. But what is to happen when all this has been achieved? Is the remainder of life to be dedicated merely to the completion and extension of his social position and his ego-consciousness? Such a point of view is certainly very widely accepted. On the other hand, we know that towards the end of the thirties, that is round about the middle of life, a curious crisis begins to make itself felt, a phenomenon which gives the lie to this one-sided extraverted attitude towards life. A patient of mine finding himself in this position brought me the following dream:

"I am with my analyst. He says to me: 'There are three aspects of wisdom to which you must pay attention; the wisdom of the positive, the wisdom of the negative, and the wisdom of daily necessity. The true art of life consists in harmonizing these three aspects of wisdom.' "

I mentioned before that life can be looked upon as a process of adaptation to pre-existing inner and outer facts, between which the small human unknown quantity must steer its course, thereby achieving maturity. This process seems to be referred to in the dream as the wisdom of daily necessity, that is the wisdom implicit in the moral choice necessitated by day-to-day decisions. The wisdom of the positive is that of the ascent and of building up, the growth of the tree of life, its enlargement and the stretching out of its branches.

But what of the wisdom of the negative? Does that imply destruction and descent in its usual negative meaning? This, however, could scarcely be described as wisdom. The expression "the wisdom of the negative" must therefore be capable of bearing another meaning. The whole of nature rests upon the double principle of growth and decay; decay, however, is not synonymous with destruction, but implies rather transformation into new growth. Decay does not mean complete death, but a dissolution of the present structure as a preliminary to its rebirth in another form. Just as in the life of a plant the first stage is governed by the principle of unfolding and expansion, so the second stage is one of in-folding and concentration. In the first stage of life all the outer organs of life are formed, whereas in the second stage the hidden growth of the fruit begins; scarcely visible from the outside, it yet contains the germ of the future plant. The fruit is, so to speak, the result and the real meaning of all the stages of development.

Looked at in this way, the wisdom of the negative no longer appears as destruction but rather as transformation into a new form. The wisdom of daily necessity is the wisdom of daily choice; it is the ego capable of the conscious experience of the great super-personal structure of life with its great and eternal opposites. The conscious choice and leadership of the ego are however limited by the fact that the ego may not neglect the great basic wisdom of the positive and negative, growth and decay, expansion and retraction, but must understand, accept and assimilate them. The first half of life is mainly dominated by the task of adaptation to the external world, implying an unfolding and expansion. The more a man has done this, and the further he has progressed in the second half of life, the more necessary does it become for him to adapt himself to the inner world, which involves a process of withdrawal and concentration. In the first half of life we may and should live without reflecting too much about life, for to live is our first duty, and by living we grow; but in the second half of life we are confronted with the need to discover the *meaning* of our life in particular and of life in general.

This problem of consciously decreasing one's outer activities in favour of an inner activity is one of the most difficult problems of the Western world. Instead of recognizing that the second half of life presents a very exacting task whose claims on the entire personality are at least as great as the claims made by the first half of life, only too many people misunderstand this period as one of merely senile resignation which they often seek to camouflage by an exaggerated busyness. Eastern culture with its profoundly introverted attitude as compared with our one-sidedly extraverted education and point of view, has far surpassed us in its understanding of the differences which distinguish the first half from the second half of life. Thus, for example, all Hindus belonging to the three upper castes consider it their duty to obey the ordinances of the four "âshramas" or the four periods of life. The first âshrama is that of the Brahmacârî, in which the disciple of the brahmans, the growing young man, must listen and learn; the second period is that of the Grihastha, the father of the family, the period of ripe manhood when a man is called upon to fulfil his social duties. These, however, are followed by the third and fourth stages, those of the Vânaprastha, the hermit, and of the Sannyâsû, the homeless beggar—duties which strike us Europeans as odd and uncanny. In India however these two last stages enshrine the specific task of the second half of life. It is no longer man's duty to pile up the goods of this world, or to fulfil the outward social duties of life, but having performed all these tasks, he must now set himself to gain the treasures of the inner world, until finally he will peacefully await his end as an anonymous beggar, so that he leaves life in the same condition of anonymity as he entered upon his earthly existence.

Such an attitude does not appear odd and still less degrading to Eastern minds; on the contrary, to them it seems the self-evident and logical development of life, and forms, therefore, an integral part of their religion. Although it would be absurd for us Western people to imitate this Eastern attitude, yet, if we understand its meaning symbolically, we shall find it very instructive. Lao-Tse expressed this attitude when he said:

> "One may know the world
> without stepping beyond one's threshold.
> One may perceive the meaning of heaven
> without looking through the window."

If a man who has already achieved his aim in the external world adopts this attitude of looking within, it will enable him to reach another level of life, thus avoiding the danger of self-stultification within the limits of the territory already conquered.

This turning-point from the positive to the negative, from the world of facts to that of the meaning, expresses itself also in our Western psychology, since the unconscious, in spite of all conscious wishes and one-sidedness, is set on achieving the state of mind necessary for the proper conduct of the second half of life. The following pictures were drawn by a man in the middle thirties who had heard the summons from the other side of life.

The first picture (cf. picture 13, page 169) is that of a coiled snake resting on top of a pool at the bottom of which a golden ball can be seen. The snake is just raising its head, and the patient felt that this meant that it was trying to reach the golden ball. The golden ball is the sun, representing the libido which is hidden in the depths of the well—the light hidden in darkness. To reach and recover it is synonymous with the process of individuation. The next picture (cf. picture 14, page 184) shows a mighty tree containing a dark door leading mysteriously into the interior. This picture forms a counterpart to the drawing by the lad of eleven which was mentioned above. The task portrayed in that picture appeared to consist in a process of growing upwards out of the root layers past the dangers threatened by the dragons, out into the light. In this case the task consists in reentering the dark womb of the earth towards the eternal mothers, along a road threatened by other dragons and other adventures than those which confronted the child.

A later picture (cf. picture 15, page 185) made by the same man was the result of a dream full of archetypal motifs. His dream was as follows: "I watched two ritual acts which followed each other, something like a sacrificial act or dance. The first ritual proceeded as a circle subdivided into four parts, and some sort of sacrifice took place in the centre. The circle originated either through a dance movement in which people approached the centre from all sides, or it was a pattern traced on the ground. For some reason this first act was only preliminary or needed another one as its completion or redemption. This second act proceeded in a kind of circular movement which was subdivided into parts."

When he awoke he felt that he had to draw this dream. He says about it: "When I did so the interaction of the two circles— the inner one in six parts and the outer one in four parts— developed immediately, with the 'altar' as centre. The altar reminded me also of a crystal. As I went on drawing there developed different layers: night- and day-sky, a water zone, two earth-layers, and a fire zone."

The clue to the dream and the drawing, which clearly belongs to the mandala-type, lies in the interaction of the two circular movements subdivided into the four and six. Jung has shown the psychological significance of the Indian Kundalini Yoga,[1] and Baynes, in his *Mythology of the Soul,* has drawn a parallel between this Eastern system of meditation and psychological integration.[2] The growing consciousness is symbolized in this system of Yoga by the rising of the serpent through seven stages of consciousness represented by seven circles or "çakras." This explains the meaning of the first picture of the snake resting on the pool. The snake is the symbol of potential consciousness, and the rising up of its head represents a first movement towards the achievement of psychological integration. In the Kundalini Yoga the lowest stage of consciousness is symbolized by a centre of çakra which is represented as a lotus flower with four petals. The next çakra is symbolized by a lotus flower with six petals. Whereas the first çakra is the "earth-çakra" where the power of consciousness is still asleep, the next one is the "water-çakra" symbolizing the fact that, when consciousness first awakens, it finds itself confronted with the power of the unconscious; and the awakening of consciousness coincides with the idea of baptism, which is a symbolical self-sacrifice according to the pattern of death and rebirth.

The dream thus points to the necessary sacrifice of an attitude which is concentrated exclusively on the concrete realities of life. The unconscious has to be accepted as the new experience —the first circular movement represented a preliminary state of consciousness, and therefore "needed another one as its completion or redemption." This is an interesting example of the power of the archetypes: how certain collective unconscious patterns are activated by psychological situations which transcend the experience of the individual, and how in those patterns a complete and satisfactory formulation of the individual crisis and an answer to it can be found.

[1] Cf. Jung, *The Integration of the Personality,* pp. 152 and 158. For a comprehensive description of the Kundalini Yoga cf. Arthur Avalon, *The Serpent Power,* Ganesh, Madras, 1924.

[2] H. G. Baynes, *Mythology of the Soul,* Bailliere, London, 1940, pp. 229ff.

The descent into the unconscious which had begun with the entrance into the dark door in the tree is taken a step further in a later drawing (cf. picture 16, page 192) which shows the patient in a little boat in the depths of the underworld. Here he is on the point of beginning his subterranean journey by passing under an arch along a dark stream lit by a midnight sun. This picture represents the archetypal motif of the "night journey under the sea,"[1] the *nekyia* or descent *ad inferos*,[2] into the depths of the unconscious, where the future solution has to be found. It is the journey to the "Western Land," to "the land of the setting sun,"[3] where "immortality," i.e. psychologically speaking integration, will be found.[4] This "Western land of the setting sun" contains a clear reference to the task of the second half of life, and thus the patient is on his way to the fulfilment of his life.

In his autobiographical volume *Rain upon Godshill*, J. B. Priestley gives a beautiful example of how the change-over from the attitude of the first half of life to that of the second half may suddenly present itself to consciousness. There he relates a dream which he had when he was forty-two.[5] He discusses the phenomenon of what he calls the "wise dream" which "seems to offer us a new and superior type of experience," and makes us feel "that for a brief while we had been attached to a mind infinitely richer and greater than our own"—a paraphrase of what Analytical Psychology would call the collective unconscious. He goes on to say: "Just before I last went to America, during the exhausting weeks when I was busy with my Time plays, I had such a dream, and I think it left a deeper impression upon my mind than any experience I had ever known before, awake or in dreams, and said more to me about this life than any book I have ever read. The setting of the dream was

---

[1] Cf. Jung, *Psychology of the Unconscious*, p. 237.
[2] Cf. Jung, *The Integration of the Personality*, p. 150.
[3] Cf. Jung, *Psychology of the Unconscious*, p. 275.
[4] The same psychological constellation is shown in the case of the man discussed above (p. 76ff.). This is also a situation typical for the change from the first to the second half of life, and correspondingly contains the motif of the *nekyia*, of the descent into the unconscious.
[5] J. B. Priestley, *Rain upon Godshill*, Macmillan, Toronto, 1939, pp. 304ff.

quite simple, and owed something to the fact that not long before my wife had visited the lighthouse here at St. Catherine's to do some bird-ringing. I dreamt I was standing at the top of a very high tower, alone, looking down upon myriads of birds all flying in one direction; every kind of bird was there, all the birds in the world. It was a noble sight, this vast aerial river of birds. But now in some mysterious fashion the gear was changed, and time speeded up, so that I saw generations of birds, watched them break their shells, flutter into life, mate, weaken, falter, and die. Wings grew only to crumble; bodies were sleek and then, in a flash, bled and shrivelled; and death struck everywhere at every second. What was the use of all this blind struggle towards life, this eager trying of wings, this hurried mating, this flight and surge, all this gigantic meaningless biological effort? As I stared down, seeming to see every creature's ignoble little history almost at a glance, I felt sick at heart. It would be better if not one of them, if not one of us all, had been born, if the struggle ceased for ever. I stood on my tower, still alone, desperately unhappy. But now the gear was changed again, and time went faster still, and it was rushing by at such a rate, that the birds could not show any movement, but were like an enormous plain sown with feathers. But along this plain, flickering through the bodies themselves, there now passed a sort of white flame, trembling, dancing, then hurrying on; and as soon as I saw it I knew that this white flame was life itself, the very quintessence of being; and then it came to me, in a rocket-burst of ecstasy, that nothing mattered, nothing could ever matter, because nothing else was real, but this quivering and hurrying lambency of being. Birds, men, or creatures not yet shaped and coloured, all were of no account except so far as this flame of life travelled through them. It left nothing to mourn over behind it; what I had thought was tragedy was mere emptiness or a shadow show; for now all real feeling was caught and purified and danced on ecstatically with the white flame of life."

For the understanding of this dream it is important to remember the fact that Priestley had worked at his Time plays, and that he was forty-two. He himself quotes the philosopher Whitehead:[1] "It is impossible to meditate on time and the creative passage of nature without an overwhelming emotion at the limitations of human intelligence." The work at the Time plays must have been such a meditation on time, and the "limitations of human intelligence" must have become obvious to him. That means, psychologically speaking, that the limitations of the individual effort as against the eternal laws of life—the limitations of the ego as against the images of the collective unconscious—presented themselves at least unconsciously to the author. The task of this particular phase of life, namely the task of consciously relating the individual to the images of the collective unconscious, had been formulated in this dream. In it "the noble sight" of "all the birds in the world," of all the ideas and activities which must be so essential to a creative man, suddenly turns into a blind, "meaningless biological effort." They reveal their preliminary character; they are legitimate in their own sphere and in their own phase of life, but at some point they become devoid of meaning. But suddenly, behind this waste and decay, a new significance, the real meaning, becomes visible. It is no longer the individual drive that matters, it is "the very quintessence of being," the "flame of life" which is revealed to the seeking eye. Life, that had become senseless in its old form, has taken on a new and incorruptible significance through being related to the more-than-personal, to the eternal flame of existence. No wonder that in describing the effect of this dream on him, Priestley goes on to say, "I had never felt before such deep happiness as I knew at the end of my dream of the tower and the birds, and if I have not kept that happiness with me, as an inner atmosphere and a sanctuary for the heart, that is because I am a weak and foolish man who allows the mad world to come trampling in, destroying every green shoot of wisdom. Nevertheless, I have not been quite the same man since. A dream had come through the multitude of business."[2]

[1] Priestley, *Rain upon Godshill*, p. 307.
[2] Ibid., p. 306.

I should like to add just one more example in order to show how the experience of the second half of life may present itself. The material is that of a woman of forty-eight who had come to me because of severe claustrophobic symptoms. The treatment soon revealed the fact that the claustrophobia was due not so much to "infantile fixations" or any particular traumatic situation—as a matter of fact the discussion of her childhood and the "reductive" analysis had played a very minor part, and had only occupied us for a very short time—but to a feeling of spiritual isolation and loss of orientation with regard to her place and purpose in life. It was mainly on that side of life that her dreams, and accordingly her analysis, had been focused.

After about seven months of intensive analysis she had a dream which impressed her deeply, and she felt the need to elaborate the dream by a process of active imagination (both the dream and the result of the active imagination will be discussed presently). The dream and the following phantasy meant the turning-point of her analysis; in them she found the answer to and the solution of her claustrophobia, and every trace of neurotic symptoms had disappeared after the discussion of the material contained in the dream and the phantasy. (It may be of interest to add that, after her symptoms had disappeared, my analysand felt nevertheless that, as her unconscious material had given her such new interest in life and had opened up such new vistas, she wanted to go on with the analysis. I willingly agreed to this as it was equally obvious to me as to her that this was no longer a case of the analytical treatment of a neurotic symptom but had developed into a genuine and creative process of integration and individuation.)

This then is the dream and the gist of the following phantasy. In the dream a man, "Mr. Prentice Jones—a correct-looking gentleman with a small attaché case; he looks as if he might be a civil servant," had disappeared in a cleft in the ground. At the place where he had disappeared, "steps have been cut in the rock, and at the bottom is a very small structure, something between a tomb and an air raid shelter, just large enough for one person." When my analysand woke up she found herself saying, "But you can't say the water doesn't exist for me while it's underground. It does exist—it's the same water."

The name "Prentice Jones" conveyed a definite meaning to her. "Jones" was just everybody, and "Prentice" stood for "apprentice." Thus "Prentice Jones" was every human being learning in the process of life. In her associations, which she had written down, she said "Mr. Prentice Jones had theoretical knowledge, but it was evidently not enough, since he was swallowed up. He no doubt had a map in his little attaché case and trusted to that; but for these explorations you want a guide and a rope. . . ." Thus she decided to "organize a rescue party for Mr. Prentice Jones" by way of active imagination. The result of this was most stimulating and resulted in the discovery of a note-book of Mr. Prentice Jones in which he had noted down his adventures from the time when he went down into the cleft, right up to the end of the expedition after he had been found by the rescue party. This note-book was also illustrated by a series of fascinating drawings. I can here give only the very beginning of the diary and the end of it.

The note-book starts as follows: "According to my map, there should be pot-holes, and perhaps caves, not far from here. I must go and see whether they really exist, and whether they correspond to my theories.—Have found a deep chasm with steps cut in the rock leading down to it. I hope it is not dangerous, but I must at any rate go a little way down.

"There is a curious structure at the bottom of the steps; it looks almost like a tomb, and yet it has an odd resemblance to one of those air raid shelters. There seems to be a kind of door. Shall I go in? I think not; it is uncanny; suppose one could not get out again? Anyway, it was for caves that I came. I wish I had the right equipment. This attaché case is cumbersome, yet I can't leave it behind."

And so he goes down. He finds himself in a big underground cave, with a large underground stream (cf. picture 17, after page

193) which comes down in an immense waterfall from a hole in the rock. Just when his candle is dying, he hears voices and is found by the rescue party, which consists of three persons: an elderly but stalwart man, with the name of Webster, who carries a lantern, a young man who is a guide with rope and axe, and a woman called Mole in whom my analysand recognized herself, between them. The guide asks him to leave his attaché case behind. "This is a great blow; must I really abandon all my notes and maps? He insists, however. I can only take this small notebook." (The four people together represent the totality of her psyche; it can be constellated when Mr. Prentice Jones's restricted consciousness has reached its limits, "when his candle is dying.")

On they go down-stream. Their adventures cover a considerable number of pages all related in Mr. Prentice Jones's notebook. (My analysand worked on this dream continuously for about six weeks.) Among other things they find an underground furnace on the top of a hill where workmen are melting gold, and a garden in which there grow metal flowers, which are "watered with the metal streams that flowed from the top of the mountain." Mole, the woman, receives one of these flowers in exchange for a spray of green leaves which had been given to her by a mysterious frog. (The appearance of a frog in dreams or phantasies frequently points to a process of transformation—a fact for which the fairy tale of the Frog Prince is a clear illustration.) A woman gardener says, "That is the one thing we have not got in this garden." She planted the spray in the earth next to a plant which had leaves of the same shape but made of yellow metal. " ' There,' she said, 'now it will grow into a tree.' She gave Mole a metal flower from the same plant."

After all kinds of further adventures, they come to a cave in the side of a great mountain.

"The entrance was low, but as soon as we were inside, we found that we were in an immense cave which looked like a cathedral; there were lofty arches and twisted columns made, I suppose, of hard, clear ice; but it might have been rock crystal. It seemed to be a natural formation; yet you might almost have thought an architect had designed it.

"We wandered for some time in the aisles of the dimly lit, natural cathedral; it was enormously lofty, but its size was not overwhelming, but on the contrary, restful; your body and mind could both move at ease in it. Presently we came to what seemed to be the central part. There was a great block of ice or crystal which looked like a high altar. In front of it there was a very large, circular mosaic pavement. It was made of innumerable small pieces of all possible colours—red, blue, green, gold, silver and purple; each piece was shaped like a flower, or a star, or a symmetrical figure of some other kind; but the whole design formed one immense flower, of a pattern so complex that it was difficult to grasp it, and yet even from what you could see you felt it was harmonious (cf. picture 19, page 225).

"Suddenly we stopped. Webster, the guide, Mole and I all saw it at the same moment—there was a gap in the mosaic pavement, of exactly the shape and size of our flower. We bent down and put the flower in its right place; it fitted exactly. 'Now the service will begin' a voice said.

"Very softly at first, but growing louder, music began. It seemed to be made of a great number of different voices, singing in complex harmonies. Some sounded like human voices and some like instruments. It was as if a great invisible congregation was singing; but also as if every pillar of the cathedral, every stone of the mountain, and every star in the sky had a voice and was singing its own tune. All the tunes made part of one great tune, just as all the flowers and stars in the pavement made one star-shaped flower.

"The guide noticed that I was writing in my book. 'What?' he said, with a smile, 'still scribbling in that note-book of yours?' But I must keep my note-book ready. For now we hear the music of the service; but perhaps later on we shall be able to hear the words.

"Then the music died away, and for a moment it was all silent.

Then, high up in the dome of the great cathedral, a single lark began singing.

"Deep down in the translucent black ice of the cathedral floor, far below the surface, there appeared a spark of light. Slowly it rose up, and grew larger; it was a ball of golden light. It came up under the very centre of the mosaic pavement; it reached the surface; the mosaic shattered into fragments with a ringing sound as it broke through the surface. As the ball of light rose higher, the scattered flowers and stars of which the pavement had been composed flew into the air and circled round it, like stars, or butterflies, or singing birds, until they seemed to dissolve in its light. Then the whole cathedral too began to dissolve; the cathedral, and the mountain in which it was enclosed, opened out like an immense flower with the globe of light at its heart. Then the flower too dissolved in light. There was nothing left but a clear blue sky with the sun shining in it; below was the earth, shining in the morning light as if it was the first day of creation.

" 'Well,' I said, 'here we are back in the daylight; and everything looks as if nothing had happened at all.'

" 'Look,' said Mole, 'here is our tree.'

"I don't know how it came to be there, but there it was: it was the green spray, and it had taken root and grown into a small tree; and on the highest branch a round, golden fruit was shining in the sun."

To go into the elaborate symbolism of this phantasy would far transcend the purpose of this essay. But even without going into details the main line is evident. Mr. Prentice Jones is truly another "Everyman" who has received the message:

> "A pilgrimage he must on him take,
> Which he in no wise may escape;
> And that he bring with him a sure reckoning
> Without delay or any tarrying."

This "correct-looking gentleman with a small attache case" finds himself engulfed in adventures "of which he would never have dreamed." He and the other two men of the rescue party represent different aspects of the animus figure. The story is another example of the *nekyia*, of the descent *ad inferos* which is so typical for this particular stage of human experience. Through different stages it leads to an extremely satisfactory answer and solution of the conflict. Her own individual flower of this earth has to be exchanged for the flower of the underworld—her individual conscious achievement is needed just as much as its eternal counterpart in the gardens of the underworld. But the climax and catharsis of the whole journey is reached when she discovers that this, her flower, fits into the grandiose mandala pattern of the mosaic pavement, when she feels that her individual life is a part and completion of a great super-individual pattern. A sense of profound harmony descends on her, until in the ecstatic experience of the golden light at the end the final answer is found. "Everything looks as if nothing had happened at all"; and yet she has found her place in life, and the knowledge of a deep significance of her individual existence, which alone gives true peace and security, has come to her. This is the real meaning of the process of individuation and integration through which she has gone.

These last examples show what are the contents and aims that must be realized and integrated in the second half of life. Whatever its precise manifestations may be, the problem posed is always one which may be described as "religious" in the widest sense of the term. It is the task of the second half of life to find an answer to the super-personal, objective meaning of life. This explains the great importance of such pictures as those of the last case, and the same obviously holds true of any dreams or visions with collective contents; they represent objective psychic contents which are not created and invented by the subject but appear to him from out of the inexhaustible plenitude of the collective unconscious. The first half of life is concerned with the development and differentiation of the ego from the background of the primeval collective images, until in the middle of life the ego has attained complete integrity.

In the first half of life, concerned as it is with the development and assertion of our own individual personality, we live as though it were we ourselves who make life, as if the experience of life were our own individual invention. And as a matter of fact, we must live in this manner; because it is only by so doing that we can achieve the consciousness of individuality and become individuals. Just because at the moment of birth our existence is quite undifferentiated from that of the collective psychic matrix, it is our necessary task to compensate for this by shaping and expressing our individual ego. As soon, however, as our ego has become strong enough, the necessity for another kind of compensation appears, namely the experience of the super-personal, super-individual layer. In the earlier phase, that of the development of the ego, all our experience was subjective, created and shaped by our subjective ego. We now have to learn that in the deepest sense we create nothing subjectively, but rather that the individual ego in virtue of its function as a receptive organ merely experiences the eternally present background of objective facts. The moment when a child first refers to itself as "I" is of cardinal importance, because this shows that it is spontaneously experiencing the fact that it is not merely identical with the world of objects which surround it. When the fully developed ego becomes aware of the images of the objective collective unconscious, it is an equally decisive moment; the ego now realizes that not every experience is subjective, but that there exists a vast psychic background whose nature it may apprehend, but which it has in no sense created.

Indeed this objective psychic background is now seen to contain the clue to the real meaning of existence. This explains the stupendous nature of all visions of God, of all those "heavenly visitations" to which, for instance, the Old Testament prophets were subject—and against which they start by putting up a resistance just because at first sight these irruptions from the unseen appear as an attack on the integrity of their own ego. And indeed the danger is very real, for if the ego, faced by these contents of the collective psychic background, is simply overwhelmed by them, its elaborately developed receptive organ is shattered and the ego is lost in a psychosis. If on the other hand the individual, owing to the strength and integrity of his subjective ego, is capable of dealing with the appearance of the objective non-ego, there is no dissolution of his personality, but instead he can, whilst realizing the subjective limits of his own ego, experience the inexhaustible wealth of the inner objective world existing beyond. The path of human development therefore leads from a condition before the ego, where the human being is still identified with the collective psychic matrix, through the stage of the ego that has separated itself from this background to a condition beyond the ego; in other words from a non-ego through an ego to a non-ego in which last stage, however, in contradistinction to the first one, the personality is capable of consciously experiencing the collective matrix. Thus our path may be said to lead from an unconscious anonymity to a conscious anonymity. It is to this last stage that Jung applies the term "self" in contradistinction to the "ego."

The way of life, therefore, leads both forwards and backwards; forwards in the direction of the maximum degree of ego-consciousness; backwards in the direction of a return to the condition of the original but now conscious unity. The figure possessing both a forward and backward inclination is the circle; he who moves forward in a circle returns to his starting-point. That is why the circle appears again and again as the symbol both of human life and eternity.

We sprang from anonymous nature and to it we must return. That does not mean that we should return to a pure state of nature, for animals and plants and stones are also pure nature, but with no conscious perception of it. To be nature with consciousness of this nature would appear to be the prerogative of man alone, who thus forms a synthesis between it and its opposite, consciousness, a synthesis which is the key to the real meaning of human existence.

"He who penetrates the great harmony of all things holds himself apart like one who is drunken with a generous wine, and who lays himself down at peace with all things. He moves in this immeasurable harmony as though he had never issued forth from the creative womb of nature. This is called the great penetration."[1]

[1]Wen-Tse (a disciple of Lao-Tse), quoted from: M. Buber, *Ekstatische Konfessionen*, Insel, Leipzig, 1921, p. 182.

V

CONSCIOUSNESS AND CURE

THERE is one question that constantly confronts every psychotherapist—a question which goes to the very root of his work: "How can you possibly expect consciousness to effect healing? We know our troubles so well, so much better than you do; how then can self-knowledge heal our wounds?"

Indeed, this question is just as important for us psychotherapists as it is for the patients. Is it the old Socratic poser: "Can virtue be taught?" masquerading in modern dress as "Can health be taught?" It would be altogether too simple to take refuge in the reply: "Wait and see; experience will show that, in fact, knowledge does bring healing." Too simple, because for one thing we ourselves must be quite clear as to the process whereby we propose to effect a cure, the process namely of becoming conscious, that is, of attaining self-knowledge; and for another, it is essential for some people that they should have some notion of what is happening or about to happen to them. It is true that if you consult a doctor about a pain in your stomach or an attack of influenza, you do not expect a discourse on his reasons for adopting this or that form of treatment. You simply trust his skill and his experience more or less blindly. But the fundamental difference between that kind of treatment and psychotherapeutic analysis is that, in physical illness, all the patient can do is to bear his sufferings more or less patiently and to follow out willingly the doctor's directions; whereas in psychotherapeutic treatment everything depends on the patient's willingness to co-operate in the fullest possible manner. Without such personal effort on the part of the patient the utmost endeavours of the psychotherapist are foredoomed to failure. An analysis makes such enormous demands on the willing co-operation of the patient's whole personality that in many cases this method is only possible, and the patient can only produce the necessary co-operation, if he fully understands the fundamental principles underlying this form of treatment and its final aim. That is why we psychotherapists have at least to try to find an answer to this question: "How can consciousness heal?"

I should like to make clear from the outset that my attempt at an answer is bound, owing to the very nature of the subject, to be theoretical and, indeed, philosophical. That is to say, I shall not proceed by heaping up examples from my practice in order to be able to say: "There, you see how knowledge (or consciousness) does in fact cure," but, taking one significant case as a basis, I shall attempt to make clear the underlying concept which renders the practical results of analytical treatment intelligible. I hope the practical importance of my theoretical disquisition will become clear.

As illustration, I will quote two dreams which a woman of forty dreamed in the course of a long analysis. She had come to me because of depressions, and a general state of anxiety. The first dream was as follows:

"A quiet lake in a forest. A black horse is grazing in a meadow alongside. After a time it becomes restless, pricks up its ears and seems to be waiting for its master. It approaches the lake in order to drink. The image reflected in the water, however, is not that of a horse but of a horseman, that is to say of a man in the position and action of riding, but without a horse. This figure is that of a handsome man in a purple cloak. The horse enters the water in order to reach the rider, whose image, however, recedes before it. The animal waits irresolutely and then trots away."

To explain all the dream's implications and peculiarities would take a long time, and I will confine myself to its salient features. The first thing that strikes one is that the horse appears to be seeking its master. The horse, as a symbol, appears constantly in myth and folklore. It is an "archetype," that is a figure emanating from the levels of the collective unconscious. The horse as an animal represents the non-human psyche, the sub-human, biological sphere, or, in psychological parlance, the unconscious. This is why in folklore horses are frequently represented as clairvoyant and clairaudient and why they sometimes even speak. The horse is also an animal that not only carries man but brings him forward, and is thus the symbol of vehicular force possessing dynamic power. "The horse is dynamic power and a means of locomotion; it carries one away like a surge of instinct. It is subject to panics like all instinctive creatures who lack higher consciousness."[1] Wotan on Sleipnir, or, considered from another aspect, those hybrid creatures the centaurs, are two examples, chosen from among countless instances, of the rôle played by the horse in mythology and folklore. The horse represents the biological libido, natural energy or, in its widest sense, the unconscious instinctual sphere. The black colour connotes the chthonic earthly side—or, to use a term of Chinese philosophy, the "Yin" side.

This primitive energy, the unconscious, requires conscious direction if it is to become productive in the human and spiritual sense. Conscious leadership is naturally represented by the rider. And that is why, in the dream, the horse is seeking its master. But it is significant that in the dream the rider is represented as the reflection of the horse itself. This indicates a truly magic relation between horse and rider. They represent a fundamental unity, but nevertheless they are separated.

The lake in the forest also represents an archetypal situation in mythology and folklore: it is the place of mystery in the sacred grove where the great transformations occur; it is the fountain of youth, the place of re-birth, of baptism, the place of initiation; it represents the unconscious fraught with magic power. In this magic field of force, the horse appears transformed into its master, representing at one and the same time both its

[1] Jung, *Modern Man in Search of a Soul*, p. 29. Cf. also Jung, *Psychology of the Unconscious*, p. 170.

own reflection and its completion on a higher level. In the dream the rider appears in the position and attitude of riding, that is as belonging to the horse and connected with him in the closest possible manner. The rider's proud bearing and mantle of royal purple indicate his exalted and dominant character. But it is clear that the horse is unable, as yet, to reach his master.

In order to understand this fact fully, we must keep in mind that the dream is dreamed by a woman. That gives the figure of the rider—a male figure—its special significance. He is a typical "animus" figure. To a woman the symbol of the man—the animus—means spirit in its widest sense; he represents the principle of Logos, as the woman in the psychology of a man— the anima—represents the principle of Eros.[1] Therefore the dream indicates to the woman that the merely instinctual, chthonic side, the unconscious, must be directed by the principle of spirit. The unconscious as the "objective psyche" must be realized and led by the subjective ego-consciousness. The rider, as representative of the spiritual principle, is still hidden in the magic waters of the lake; he is only an immaterialized reflection, that is an unrealized idea, and must first be born from the deep waters of the unconscious, teeming with life. At present the horse is unable to reach the rider, and the closer it comes the further its master's image recedes. An unknown power prevents these two components of what is, after all, an essential unity from meeting.

This dream proceeds from the deepest levels of the unconscious. The unconscious psyche has not yet been sufficiently prepared and the higher level of consciousness represented by the unity of rider and horse cannot, therefore, as yet be attained; the unknown force separating the two is still too strong. This power must first be robbed of its harmful effect; that is it must be recognized for what it is, before the great act of union can take place, and the ultimate, spiritually pre-destined unity can be achieved. The practical therapeutic problem is, of course, the nature of this hidden fact which makes union impossible. In

[1] Cf. Jung: "Woman in Europe," in *Contributions to Analytical Psychology*.

order to answer this question it is necessary to study the dream which immediately followed the first. The second dream was as follows:

"I was in a large, beautiful ante-room, built in the classical style. Although there was a good deal of open space between the pillars, there was no view as the view was entirely blocked by hanging rugs. The space between the two middle pillars was filled in by a beautiful soft blue-grey kangaroo skin. I knew that it was from between these two pillars that the sources of the Nile should gush out, and I was longing to see them burst forth. I attempted to drag away the skin but it was so firmly attached that this was impossible. It was only in my mind's eye that I could see the waters flow."

Obviously the central symbol is the kangaroo skin blocking up the sources of the Nile. Our spontaneous reaction is a feeling that the sources of the Nile should flow freely, a feeling which also finds expression in the words and actions of the dreamer. It is quite clear that, in spite of its beauty, the skin plays a negative rôle, inasmuch as it blocks up the sources of the Nile. As for the symbolical meaning of the Nile, it is proverbially noted for its fertilizing power.

Without any knowledge whatsoever of the patient's associations we are able to interpret the dream as pointing to a condition in which a human being is prevented from making full use of his living, active and creative powers by something which, although in itself beautiful and valuable, is yet in this connection exerting an inhibiting effect. This general impression is confirmed and intensified when we come to consider the circumstances and associations of the dreamer.

She was a handsome German woman who looked considerably younger than her forty years, the mother of two obviously gifted and attractive children, who gave her life its meaning and content. Her husband had died a few years previously. To find out the causes of her anxiety and depression, I had asked her to tell me the story of her life, with special reference to her marriage. Everything appeared to have been in order and, according to her account, she had lived on the happiest and most harmonious terms with her husband, who had been a very distinguished doctor and scientist. She herself, before and immediately after the outbreak of the first world war, had been a medical student, and it was at the university that she had got to know her future husband. From all she told me, and indeed from all I could gather in other ways, her husband had been not only an eminent scientist, but also a most devoted and kindly human being, and she had in addition every reason to be proud of her two children. Moreover, her financial circumstances were assured, so that the only external cause to account for her depression was, apparently, the loss of her husband about five years previously. Oddly enough, however, she always strenuously denied this very obvious suggestion. She admitted willingly that she had suffered deeply and was still suffering from his loss, but she was absolutely convinced that this was not the cause of her neurosis, more especially as she now remembered that even during her marriage she had suffered from similar, apparently causeless and quite inexplicable, attacks.

Faced with such a situation every experienced observer will, in spite of the patient's obvious sincerity and apparent justification, view with a certain suspicion her assurances that the matrimonial horizon was absolutely unclouded. Moreover, analysis gradually revealed the fact that my patient's husband was almost completely absorbed in his work and that he made great claims on his wife's help and support, both inwardly and outwardly, so that she had very little time left "for herself." In spite of this she repeated again and again that she had accepted this state of things without the slightest feeling of being coerced. Progress in this direction seemed, therefore, impossible. Although from all she told me I had some notion of the line our enquiry would ultimately take, namely that of the suppression of her own individuality and personal development, she was not ready to accept my suggestion, so that *my* knowledge would have been of no help to her. It was at this juncture that this dream made its dramatic appearance. When she told me the dream, the obvious thing to do was to enquire further about the striking kangaroo skin. At first she could tell me nothing about it. But at last it suddenly occurred to her that she had seen this very kangaroo skin twenty years before in the house of her mother-in-law. Once the ice was broken she told me, with considerable emotion, the following story:

Shortly before the outbreak of war in 1914 a young English doctor was working at the university where she was studying medicine. The two became very friendly, and eventually fell deeply in love with each other. They were just about to become engaged when war broke out, and the abrupt departure of her English friend put an end to all these beautiful plans. Meanwhile she had, during her student days and concurrently with her attachment to the young Englishman, formed a friendship with her future husband, who held an appointment at the same hospital. He fell in love with her and made her an offer of marriage. Although she liked him well enough, she had at first refused his offer, as she intended to marry the Englishman, but in the difficult situation in which she found herself, she agreed, not without considerable inner conflict, to become engaged to the German. Her inner resistance finally became so strong that she decided, in spite of all her liking and sympathy for her fiancé, to break her engagement. With this purpose in view, she took the train to another town where her fiancé happened to be staying with his mother. As she entered the house of her future mother-in-law, the first thing she saw was an enormous kangaroo skin, which had a peculiar connection with her fiancé. In his scientific capacity, he had been commissioned by the directors of a large Zoological Garden to carry out post-mortems on their deceased animals. In this way the kangaroo skin had come into his possession, and he gave it to his mother. What happened on this visit was that my patient was so overwhelmed by the affectionate greetings of her mother-in-law and by pity for her fiancé, that she felt unable to carry out her original intention of breaking off her

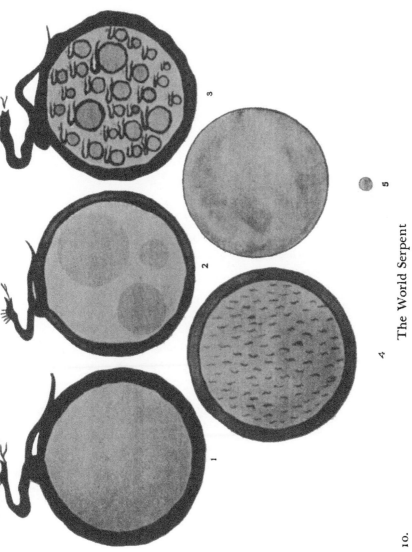

The World Serpent

10.

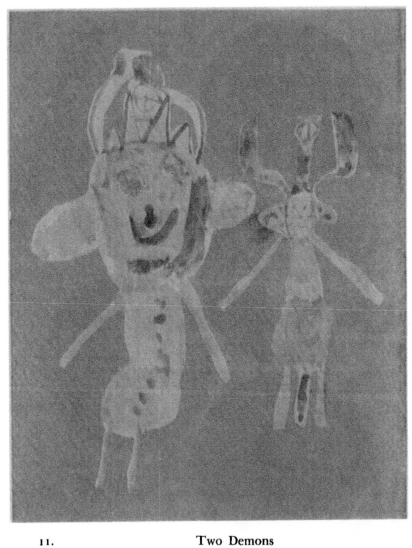

11.   Two Demons

engagement, and only succeeded in binding herself to him even more closely, with the result that she very soon married him. In the course of her harmonious and, on the whole, very happy married life, she had managed to repress all this, and consequently she also managed to forget completely the existence of the kangaroo skin. Nevertheless, her unconscious mind retained the image and, because of its striking and impressive appearance, and above all because it was the first thing that struck her in the home of her mother-in-law, where such momentous events took place, the kangaroo skin became, so to speak, the symbol for her equivocal decision about her marriage.

This story provided an opportunity for getting at the meaning of the dream. Considering it from the purely reductive aspect—that is, relating its contents to a repressed experience—the marriage problem obviously occupies the central position. Just as the kangaroo skin had dammed back the accumulated waters of the Nile, and prevented their flow along their natural channels, so my patient's marriage had put a stop to the development of her own personal life and individual abilities. She had obviously made a heroic attempt to suppress her dimly-felt knowledge of having made a mistake, by subordinating herself entirely to the interests and personality of her kindly and gifted husband, at the cost however of completely losing her own line of life. The seriousness of the resultant split and the degree of her resistance to any conscious admission of the real state of things can be gauged by the fact not only that she should be able to forget so completely such a remarkable object as the kangaroo skin, but that it should require such concentrated effort on her part to reconstruct its history.

Actually, of course, it is precisely the existence of such strong resistances which explains why, in this and similar cases, the true state of things can only be unravelled with the help of an analysis. The aim of analysis is, so to speak, to free a passage for the dammed-up waters by helping to remove the kangaroo skin which was blocking their outlet. However vehemently my patient had previously refused to accept my suggestion that her marriage might to some extent account for her difficulties, she could not deny the facts of her dream.

To confine the meaning of the dream to a mistaken decision made twenty years ago would, however, be altogether too one-sided and would completely fail to do justice to its compensatory and constructive character. No doubt this mistaken decision had hampered my patient's inner development very considerably, but it must not be forgotten that, in spite of this, her marriage had been very happy and had consequently provided her with sufficient positive values to compensate for its more doubtful aspects. It is therefore necessary to enquire why the dream should choose this precise moment to recall to memory an event which had happened so long ago; in other words, what is its significance in her actual situation?

Dreams function with supreme economy; if a dream reproduces a situation belonging to the remote past it is because of its bearing on the present. Granted that the recognition and acceptance of a repressed experience is in itself an important factor for good, one is nevertheless bound to ask in what way it is going to help this poor woman in her present distress to realize that she committed a cardinal error all those years ago. Will it not rather exacerbate her anxiety neurosis by leading her to doubt the value of her previous life and achievements? If the recognition of past mistakes is to be valuable, in other words productive, it must contain a hint as to how the error can be rectified and so conduce to a better life in the future. This is the constructive and synthetic aspect of a dream in contradistinction to its reductive and analytical aspect. This constructive aspect is immediately seen if the mistake, as revealed in the dream, is understood to refer not only to one isolated instance in the past but is considered typical and symptomatic of the patient's whole attitude to life. The dream disclosed a difficult situation in which my patient had acted against her "better judgment" and allowed herself to be fatally influenced and led by the wishes and needs of others instead of pursuing the path which she herself instinctively knew to be the right one. She had submitted passively to the influence of others instead of actively shaping her own life. In other words, she had adopted a typically one-sided feminine attitude.

It is significant that this same problem was adumbrated in the preceding dream of the horse and rider. This dream revealed the necessity of correcting and supplementing the purely feminine and instinctive side of her nature by conscious control through the intellectual or masculine principle, thus lifting her whole life on to a higher level.[1] The dream also implied that this fusion of forces was opposed by certain subterranean influences. It is only with this in mind that the true meaning of the dream of the blocked sources of the Nile becomes apparent. The dream is a parable of her *present* psychological situation and duties. It stands to reason that if an intelligent and gifted woman of forty is entirely sunk in memories of the past and the care of her children, she is seriously neglecting the duty of developing her own spiritual personality. Her development has been arrested by becoming fixed in a typically feminine and passive attitude to life, and she must learn to compensate for this by adopting a more active "masculine" attitude. The kangaroo dream recalls to mind her previous mistake as a warning in her present difficulties, where similar influences are still at work threatening to block the outflow of living water.

The compensating attitude, which must be adopted if the waters are to flow once more, is symbolized in the first dream by the figure of the rider. He represents the active, courageous, masculine attitude of self-confident leadership as opposed to that of passive subjection. The dream of the horse and rider, therefore, sets out as it were a plan of campaign. It is significant that in this dream-plan horse and rider are unable as yet to meet; indeed for the moment the rider is not even actually,

[1]It is essential to avoid the mistaken assumption that the masculine principle is in itself superior to the feminine. Each is compensatory to the other. Thus, a man who has lived a too one-sided, masculine life—e.g. an intellectual and active one—needs to compensate by developing a more "feminine" attitude, e.g. through a development of his feeling side. Equally, a too-feminine woman needs to develop her intellectual side. Completion can only be achieved by the synthesis of Logos and Eros.

but merely potentially, present. This still unrealized conception—whose realization is nevertheless essential if my patient is to overcome her depression and disorientation—is that compensating element in feminine psychology of which she is still quite unconscious, namely the masculine spiritual principle as it is personified in the figure of the animus; whereas she has stuck fast in a purely instinctive and outworn feminine attitude. The first step towards the adoption of a more active and vigorous way of life will naturally be to acknowledge her previously repressed conviction as to what she should have done. That is why the dream brings back to consciousness a situation which she had repressed, and it is just because the obligations associated with this admission of error are so difficult and critical for her, as a woman, with a woman's feelings and ideals, to accept, that she must first take this step if she is to find a new adaptation to life which will make a cure possible. That is why the dream reveals her typical attitude to life. As soon, however, as she begins to accept this knowledge and these obligations and to incorporate·them into life (i.e. to assimilate the knowledge she has gained), the hitherto unsubstantial figure of the rider materializes, and horse and rider can come together.[1]

It is evident that the separation of horse and rider, as shown in the dream, indicates a split in the mind of the dreamer and an unsatisfied and unresolved state of tension. And it is equally evident that my patient's depression and state of anxiety can only be cured when this split is bridged, or, to use the phraseology of the dream, when horse and rider come together. I should like to pursue the implications of the dream still further,

---

[1] In actual fact the two dreams discussed above formed the pivotal point of the subsequent treatment. Further analysis made it clearer and clearer that the neurotic symptoms had been due to the neglect and retardation of her individual development. From a dependent and undecided person the patient turned into an active and independent woman who could shape her life according to her needs. Thus for instance she built up a new career for herself, based on her former medical training, in which she found an adequate and satisfactory outlet for her energies. Moreover, new and unexpected human relationships opened up for her which corresponded to her nature and furthered her spiritual development. To her it appeared as if she lived in a changed world; but it was really in herself that the change had taken place.

and, basing myself on this condition of cleavage, find an answer to the question posed at the outset, viz. in what way knowledge, and what kind of knowledge, can bring about a cure. We have already seen that horse and rider symbolize instinctual energy on the one hand and conscious leadership on the other. They also represent something else, something on a higher level and of much deeper significance, for, taken in conjunction, they symbolize a certain inseparable whole. They form a unity complete in itself, irrespective of the significance of its component parts. The horse is an entity in itself and the rider is an entity in himself, and yet the significance of the dream lies in the fact that, although these two pictures exist side by side, each component achieves its full and essential meaning only when the other component has joined up with it: each half presupposes the other. In this connection horse implies a rider, just as the term ruler implies the ruled, or as right is incomplete without left, or North without South; or, to use a Chinese symbol, Yang and Yin are inseparably intermingled. One part in the absence of the other is, in its deepest meaning, unfinished and in need of completion. Both parts possess a meaning of their own, but both together connote something other and greater than the mere sum of their separate entities; horse plus rider, ruler plus people, Yang plus Yin: something other and greater than their sum, namely the union of the two, an indestructible unity which is actually conditioned by their mutual interdependence. It is not just a question of any given horse and of some independent and, so to speak, casual man who happens to come along, but rather of a pre-existing mutual relationship: the horse is seeking *his* master, the rider belongs to *his* horse.

It is precisely this relationship which constitutes a dynamic force, i.e. when one component is posited the other immediately springs to mind, even if it only exists as latent energy. And it is precisely when this state of dynamic tension occurs and each component is straining to join its other half that the critical moment has arrived when consciousness will produce a cure. Whenever the dynamic tension appears, and an incomplete half conjures up, because of its very incompleteness, its other component element, it summons into existence the inevitable urge for completeness, for "wholeness." When the dream evokes the image of the horse, it predicates the inevitable and obvious figure of the rider. As long as the one exists without the other, so long does it remain the unsatisfied and therefore of necessity the seeking partner. To become conscious is, therefore, to become aware of the other half, to acquire knowledge of the part that is missing. Consciousness consists in taking possession, through knowledge, of a pre-determined whole. Only when the missing part has been assimilated into consciousness is the desire for wholeness satisfied and at rest; only then is the negative state of tension resolved. This is the crux of the matter.

There is inherent in man a longing and tendency towards wholeness, and only when this longing is stilled is his negative state of tension wiped out and neutralized. This wholeness can only be achieved through knowledge of the missing part, that is when a man has become fully conscious. That is what is meant, for instance, by the sentence in the Upanishads: "Brahma is the knowledge of Brahma."

In that magnificent myth in the *Symposium,* Plato speaks of the earlier state of mankind, when their nature was still androgynous, that is both male and female, and they were quite round like a ball. Each human being had four hands and four feet, two faces supported by one neck; one head between the two faces, with four ears; the private parts were double and so was everything else. Great and terrible was their might, daring them to scale the very heavens and lay sacrilegious hands upon the gods. To punish them for their insolent temerity, Zeus decided to split them in two—so that henceforth they walked on two legs. But ever since, each half of the original man longs passionately for his other half, and if they come together they throw their arms about one another, seeking to grow into one. From this time onwards Eros was implanted in the hearts of men, striving ever to bring them back to their original state, and to make of twain one being, and so bring healing to their riven nature. As of old, two friends on parting would split a dice in two, whereby they might recognize each other in years to come, so each man is but half a dice, ever seeking his other half.

The symbolism of this story from Plato is immediately apparent, but I would like to consider it a little more closely from the psychological aspect. Eros is represented as the great instigator of unrest; Eros is the urge towards completeness, and it is indeed through Eros that we experience the creative unrest which drives each human being out of the circumscribed limits of his own life and makes him experience his other half, be this male or female. It is as if this experience necessarily and inevitably calls forth what may be described as an inherent desire for wholeness; or, to use the words of Plato: "This striving for wholeness is therefore the work of Eros."

Now this innate striving for wholeness is the decisive factor in any real understanding of the process whereby healing is brought about by consciousness. In every psychic system, every psychic organism, as found in every individual, there exists this inherent desire for completeness, which, making use of the life process, does its utmost to force him to realize this latent conception of wholeness, whether we give the resultant sum total the name of "character" or "personality." Whenever in any given life this unity or wholeness is not in process of being achieved the particular meaning and purpose of that life has gone astray. This idea is as old as the hills and is found both in the East and the West. Thus the Upanishads say: "He who leaves this world without having recognized his true world, has as little profit therefrom, owing to his failure in understanding, as he would have from the Vedas which he had not studied, or from a task which he had neglected to perform."[1]

In Europe, Aristotle was the first to work out this idea in all its implications, in his conception of "entelechy." Entelechy means literally "that which carries in itself its goal." This means that all living matter contains in itself a certain principle which strives

[1]Brihadâranyaka Upanishad, I, 4.

to mould it until it has attained a certain shape already predestined for it by this very principle. Entelechy is the energy which transforms the potential into the actual and in this way brings living matter to its perfection, the goal of its being. The pip of an apple, an acorn or the egg of a butterfly contain more or less undifferentiated matter, for the time being still formless, but nevertheless out of this structureless matter results nothing less than an apple tree, an oak or a butterfly. We have all witnessed these phenomena so often that we are only too apt to disregard the incomprehensible marvel they conceal and in part reveal. What Aristotle means by entelechy is precisely this incomprehensible, marvelous tendency of differentiation which is revealed when undifferentiated matter assumes in the course of its development its unique and predestined form.

It seems that the principle which has just been illustrated by a few examples from biology is just as active in human psychology. It is the life principle of each individual; it is, in other words, the principle of individuation. This means that every human being possesses a latent wholeness, an entity which it is possible for him to realize and which it is his life's work to realize, just as though it had been mapped out for him in the stars at his birth. This predestined form remains at first only latent, and acts as a force driving all men in a given direction. Life itself, with all the experiences and duties which must be met, strives to make man fulfil his own individual task.

At first a child cannot be called an individual; his actions and reactions are largely conditioned by his environment, and he remains identified with his parents. In the course of time, however, this natural identity with his parents must be progressively resolved in order to achieve an individual attitude to life. When this does not take place the growing youth remains too much tied to his parents and therein lies one of the commonest causes why human beings make wrong decisions. Such parent fixation may show itself in many ways. For instance, a son may adopt a profession not because he really wishes to or because of any special aptitude for it, but because of his father,

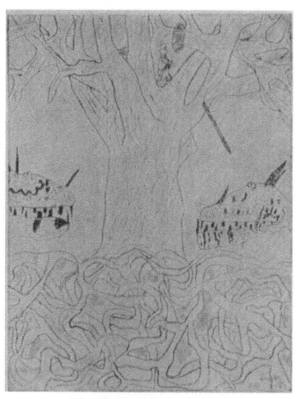

12.   The Fight with the Dragons

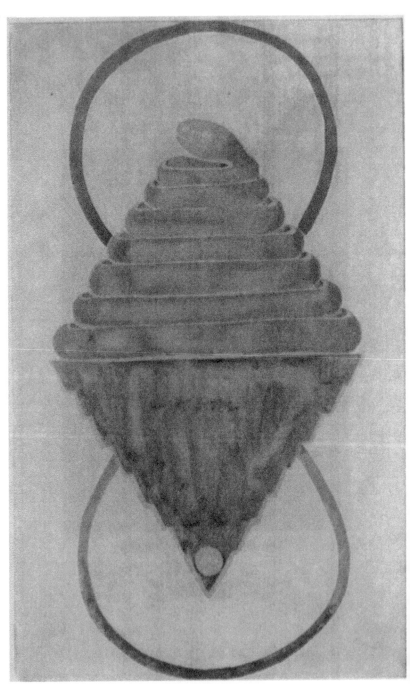

The Snake Pool

who in spite of a strong leaning towards such a profession, himself had been unable to take it up; or a daughter may marry a man who really corresponds to her mother's "type," and so on. But the common denominator in all cases is the fact that a man is measuring life by other standards than those which are natural to him and consequently he never looks at things with his own eyes. Thus he never attempts to solve a problem on his personal responsibility—be it a question of personal relationship, of choice of a profession, or of religious or intellectual problems.

When, however, the growth of the individual in personal responsibility proceeds unhindered and undisturbed a neurosis will not develop. Spiritual wrestlings and conflicts betoken man's struggle to get through towards an ever closer approximation to his real self, and individual growth is neither stultified nor arrested. In such a case, to use the words of the dream, the waters of the Nile flow freely, and there exists no obstruction which hinders the river from gushing forth on its life-giving mission. But psychotherapists unfortunately know only too well that this unhindered rush and flow of the waters of life is the exception, and that in most cases the source has been more or less blocked up, and laborious cleansing operations have to be undertaken before the water can once more stream forth unhindered. The neurosis consists precisely in this damming up, this estrangement from the real self.

Let us consider a neurosis from this point of view. It is well known that psychic energy deprived of its proper outlet becomes perverted, and instead of functioning in a progressive and constructive manner develops regressive and destructive tendencies; just as a river, when its natural outflow is obstructed, overflows its banks, bringing widespread havoc and disaster in its train. A child whose spontaneous psychic reactions are thwarted becomes stubborn and aggressive, or else reacts with fears and an exaggerated helplessness. If an adult lives a life contrary to his real nature, whether by pressure of external circumstances or from some inner motive, he is similarly crippled, and develops a neurosis. The feeling of fear—be it conscious or unconscious—is an integral component of every neurosis, whatever shape the neurosis itself may assume. The words anxiety and anguish are etymologically derived from the Latin word "angere," to throttle or choke. Such anxiety or dread is a fear of being hemmed in, of living in such confinement that there is danger of suffocation. Fear is the inevitable accompaniment of a feeling of suffocation. The function of air in the physical sphere has its exact counterpart in the psychic sphere: fear is the feeling of being cut off from something that is absolutely necessary to life.

This feeling of being separated from something essential was expressed for instance in the dream of the rider and his horse, where the two component parts were separated; and this corresponded with the feelings of anxiety shown by the patient in real life. One could define the feeling of fear which crops up in every neurosis as an instinctive feeling of being separated from one's own essential needs; or a feeling of discrepancy between actual life and life as it should be lived. The tragic element in this fear is that it grows by what it feeds on, a process which is only too familiar in psychology as the magnetic power of a complex. Thus this feeling of being separated from the main stream of life only intensifies the tendency towards self-protection, resulting in an increased withdrawal from life. Fear, therefore, always acts as a regressive force, inasmuch as it plunges a man still deeper into his own isolation, so that in the end he finishes up in a complete cul-de-sac.

The positive counterpart of anxiety or dread, however, is longing. Dread connotes a feeling of something lacking, and this feeling leads a man to flee from the claims which are made on him. Longing is also a feeling of something lacking but in the opposite sense, inasmuch as longing drives a man to try to obtain that which he lacks. In this way longing, in contradistinction to fear, urges a man to achieve his desire. This seems to me to be the psychological meaning of the platonic idea of Eros. In Plato's story Eros arises from a lack in nature, which expresses itself in longing; longing, of course, for completion. So Eros embodies a striving towards wholeness: the longing of the soul to encompass its true end and purpose. That is why Plato speaks of Eros as the great Daimon, the messenger of the gods, the saviour, who stands midway and bridges the chasm separating mortals and immortals; I should like to interpret this as the bridge linking the idea and the reality. Eros, the longing aroused by the feeling of insufficiency, is the spur, the impulse, the motive power. Fear, aroused by the feeling of insufficiency, has a paralysing effect, resulting in isolation and a crippling of man's powers. In the last resort, the task of an analysis is to liberate this positive force Eros from the negative toils of fear; for, however strange this may appear, both are but different manifestations of the same psychic energy, the libido.

The very fact that fear is the negative aspect of Eros explains why every neurosis also produces to some extent a break with society and human fellowship, and in particular with the society of the opposite sex. Individuation must not, therefore, be taken as in any sense implying an egotistical life, a life apart, but it forms on the contrary the basis of all true relationship and integration within the human society.

Of course, there are many people who seem to be missing the true meaning of their lives without apparently suffering from any neurosis. The explanation of such cases is that the resultant fear has been, so to speak, crystallized and encapsulated. It is thus rendered seemingly harmless, but the negative aspect of this unconscious process is that the encapsulated energy must be withdrawn from the stream of life and acts therefore as a minus quantity; so that all such people live with only a fraction of the energy which was their birthright. They may therefore be said to lead only half a life, or even less. This is also the explanation of the resistance exhibited by such people towards an analysis, for analysis would force them not only to realize that they have taken the wrong road, but also to face the very existence of the fears which they have so carefully hidden away under lock and key.

Considered from this point of view, a neurosis represents the last convulsive effort of the psyche to reach a positive solution, inasmuch as it gives a man no peace and drives him into such a state of unrest and dissatisfaction that at last his need to escape from the bonds of fear becomes stronger than all the negative forces. That is why the psychotherapist often finds that some of the potentially most valuable human beings come to him for help, because their neurosis, with all its fear and anguish, nevertheless acts as a spur driving them to overcome the obstacle which is alienating them from their real being, and enabling them to reach their true destination. Only that man is afraid of life who is not living as he should live. For, in the last resort, the element of fear in a neurosis is due to the very split which prevents a man from realizing his true personality, and this breach can only be healed by his adopting a new orientation towards life.

Therefore, in the end, consciousness, or better still, the process of becoming conscious, always implies becoming aware of one's real personality and of its predestined wholeness. It is as if there were a central image, an *eidos*, working behind all manifestations of life and determining them. The wholeness is achieved—in other words the entelechy has been fulfilled—in proportion as the central image, the eidos, determines every single act of the personality, and finds therein its full and undisturbed actualization.

There is an obvious difference between the purely biological and the psychological wholeness. With plants and animals—and to a relatively large extent also with primitive people and children—the actualization of the eidos is more or less achieved; they present an organic and unbroken wholeness. This explains their natural "beauty" and undisturbed rhythm. This beauty, however, is purely instinctive, "unconscious"; it might be described as belonging purely to the aesthetic sphere. With man a completely new factor enters the situation which disturbs the instinctive wholeness: it is that of consciousness and with it discrimination and choice. An animal or a plant—and to a lesser degree a primitive or a child—is unconsciously whole. With consciousness this instinctive wholeness is at first lost. Man can actualize his *a priori* "human" wholeness only in and through continuously repeated acts of choice and decision. The eidos of wholeness is present in him all the time, but it is not automatically and instinctively actualized as it is in the sphere of biological wholeness. As a matter of fact, the factor of conscious choice, of deliberate decision is the constituent element of human wholeness. The freedom of the individual might be defined as the preparedness to be formed by his own eidos, his inner image of wholeness which exists *a priori* in him. The more the individual becomes sensitive and receptive to this inner image, the more he becomes whole and "healed." The fact that language has one root for the words "whole," "holy" and to "heal" conceals a deep truth; he who is whole is also healed; to be healed is to be made whole. And it is just because this predestined, unique "wholeness," which is called personality,[1] is the real meaning and purpose of each life, that consciousness of this wholeness produces healing. It is "holy" in as far as it represents a profound experience of a numinous character; the idea of wholeness is, in other words, an archetype of deep significance. This wholeness as a predestined constellation is latent in every man and awaits its realization. Thus individuation implies a "coming to oneself." That is why the recognition of one's true self obliterates the cleavage and its accompanying fear. It is precisely this problem of wholeness which finds its expression in the dream of the horse and rider.

At the same time the integrated personality does not merely express the *individual* totality, for in the actualization of his own *a priori* wholeness the individual also discovers his relatedness to a super-individual centre. This centre is the self which is "paradoxically the quintessence of the individuum and at the same time of the collectivum."[2] In other words: the experience

[1]The Shorter Oxford English Dictionary defines "personality" as "distinctive individual character especially when of a marked kind."
[2]Jung, *Paracelsica*, p. 167.

of wholeness coincides with the experience of a centre of the personality and a meaning of life which transcends the individual. This is expressed for instance in the words of Nicolaus of Cusa who makes God say to man: *"Sis tus tuus, et ego ero tuus"*[1]—"be thou thyself, and I shall be thine."

Symbols like those of the rider and his horse are a first glimpse of this distant aim of wholeness. In them an idea is expressed which at present considerably transcends the level of consciousness, but at the same time acts as a signpost and as a directing force. The process of individuation of which they are a manifestation often appears to be an almost involuntary process, i.e. one in which the self tries to assert itself against the limited and limiting ideas and complexes, fears and desires of the ego. From this angle the psychological process of life appears as the creative expression of the tension between two poles: on the one hand the empirical ego, the personality as given here and now, and on the other hand the self, the final and eternal eidos of wholeness, of the *"homo totus."* This explains why we may have dreams or visions which transcend our present understanding and often only reveal their meaning years later. The psychic process takes place on many different levels at once and reveals its meaning according to the level which our present empirical ego has reached. Thus a symbol has a different meaning according to whether it is looked at from the empirical now and here or from the ideal self, as the final aim of the process of individuation. In this sense our physical conception of time and causality has almost to be reversed for an understanding of the psychic process: it is not the "before" in time which explains the "after" in the psychological development, but it is the psychic "after," the self, which explains the psychic processes which take place "before," that is until the wholeness is more or less realized. The psychic "after," the final power of the self in us, determines the experiences of the ego to a large extent; according to our individuality and to the degree to

[1]Quoted from Toni Wolff, *Einführung in die Grundlagen der Komplexen Psychologie*, p. 30.

which the empirical ego has integrated the eidos, our reaction to one and the same object is different. The more the ego becomes open to the influence of this eidos in himself, of the self, the further the process of individuation can progress.

It is thus the self which is the real power behind the manifestations of our psychic life, and which is the urge towards consciousness and wholeness. It manifests itself even in the neurosis; that is as a compensating and correcting psychic force where the individual has lost his bearings. Until the empirical ego, the instrument of realization, has achieved maturity in the solution of the concrete problems of life, until the facts and tasks of practical life have been accepted, the self is far beyond reach. In the acceptance and fulfilment of the here and now, of concrete reality, the reach of our consciousness is enlarged step by step. Only a consciousness that grows and matures thus in the fulfilment of life can be an equal partner to the symbolical side of life. (Psychotic people, for example, may produce the profoundest symbols, but they are unable to integrate them owing to this very lack of an ego-consciousness.) If, on the one hand, the image of the self is the power in the future which shapes our experiences in the present, it is the ego on the other hand which has to approach the unconscious and thus to discover the different and ever-growing meanings of the symbol.

Consider the dream of the sources of the Nile: until the acute problems of relationship and life, with all their necessities and failures, are known and faced, the symbol of wholeness as it is expressed in the first dream cannot reveal its constructive energy. Through the neurotic symptoms the individual is forced to take the first step towards a re-orientation, and as long as the difficulties of concrete life are not accepted and solved, no healing and no wholeness is possible. But it is this very necessity of absolute honesty towards oneself that makes analysis the deepest and most searching form of treatment to which it is possible to submit; for, in the last resort, it is an attempt to contact the self, and is thus an appeal to man's highest moral and ethical nature.

VI

A PSYCHOLOGICAL APPROACH
TO RELIGION

I

AN ATTEMPT at a psychological approach to religion is open
to misunderstandings both from the side of religion and from
that of psychology. Both the religious thinker and the psychologist may regard religion and psychology as incompatible,
though for diametrically opposite reasons. To the religious
thinker it may appear almost sacrilegious to approach the highest
content of religion—God—with the "dissecting knife" of psychology. To anyone who holds this view it must, however, be
pointed out that religion is most certainly a phenomenon of the
human psyche, and as such open to psychological enquiry. It
would indeed be a sacrilege if, in the course of its investigation,
psychology claimed to be able to make any statement about the
absolute existence or non-existence of God, or about any other
reality of religious faith. It is not the task of psychology to make
such statements, and if it did so it would clearly transcend its
competence and possibilities: the realities of faith are, as such,
not accessible to psychology. What is, however, the legitimate
concern of psychology is the *phenomenon* of religious experience
as an activity of the human psyche and as an expression of its
inner processes. Psychology is thus not concerned with the question of the reality of God, but with a psychic experience which is
understood to be and formulated as God. This experience may
or may not correspond to the existence of an absolute Deity;
but in any case it is a *psychic reality* of the greatest importance.
On this understanding, psychology does not touch the con-

ceptions of religion and theology which are based on faith in the absolute reality of God. It is only concerned with the appearance that this religious reality takes on in the human mind. In other words, psychology is concerned with ideas as they manifest themselves in the human psyche. It is thus a "misunderstanding that the psychological treatment or explanation reduced God to nothing but psychology. It is, however, not a matter of God but of ideas of God. . . . It is man who has such ideas and creates for himself images, and these things belong to psychology."[1] Psychology accepts these ideas and images of God as *psychic realities*, but cannot go into the question of the *absolute reality* behind them, which is the concern of religion.

On the other hand, to many psychologists religion seems hardly worth investigation, because they regard it as merely an "epiphenomenon." According to this view, religion is a mere concomitant of some primary biological instinct, and is one of many possible sublimations of it. For example, the two other great schools of modern "depth-psychology," those of Sigmund Freud and of Alfred Adler, would both tend to reduce religious phenomena to something else. In accordance with the fundamental conception of these two schools, this something else is, in the former case, an escape from or a sublimation of the sex instinct, and, in the latter, an instrument in the fight for superiority. In other words, to them religion—and the same remark applies to their conception of art—is at best no more than a kind of secondary psychic activity originating in the repression of some primary biological instinct. Religion is therefore nothing but a substitute for something else and loses all importance as a phenomenon *per se;* it is only worthy of study as an instance of the mechanism of repression of infantile sexuality or an infantile drive for power. The psychologist who does not accept this valuation—or rather devaluation—of religion is regarded with suspicion as introducing metaphysical or mystical elements into the realm of psychology. (It is of course this purely reductive line

[1] Jung, *Zur Psychologie der Trinitätsidee.* In: Eranos Jahr-Buch 1940–1941, Zürich, 1942, p. 50, n.1.

of argument which has turned religious thinkers against any sort of psychological interpretation of religious phenomena.)

Against this line of argument it must be pointed out that it is a thoroughly unproven assumption that religious experiences are due to "nothing but" repressions of sexual or other biological instincts. "The unconscious is a living, and therefore creative, process, and . . . it does not need any pathological repression to release its creative functions."[1] Spirituality is not a derivative of some other instinct; on the contrary, it is a primary function of the psyche, i.e. it is "a principle *sui generis,* an indispensable form of instinctual power."[2] Religious activity is the highest form of spirituality; religious phenomena are therefore not a sublimation of or an escape from something else, but expressions of an authentic and genuine function of the human psyche existing in its own right. Thus the study of religious experience is the study of a fundamental psychic process which cannot be investigated through any other phenomena. The psychological exploration of religion is not only full of interest for the psychologist, but is absolutely indispensable if he wants to do justice to the psychic process in all its fullness. This, by the way, was exactly the point at which Jung originally parted company with Freud. In his *Psychology of the Unconscious,* which appeared in 1912, he showed that the libido had a dichotomous way, namely that of instinctual processes (in the narrower sense of the biological instincts) and that of spiritual processes, whereas Freud adhered to his view that spiritual processes were merely derivatives of instinctual ones.

It goes without saying that psychological study of religious phenomena in the human psyche must obey the rules of psychological exploration. Jung has put this point very clearly in the following passage: ". . . the methodological standpoint of that kind of psychology which I represent . . . is exclusively phenomenological, that is, it is concerned with occurrences, events, experiences, in a word, with facts. Its truth is a fact and not a

---

[1] Jung, *Contributions to Analytical Psychology,* p. 364.
[2] Ibid., p. 66.

judgment. Speaking for instance of the motive of the virgin birth, psychology is only concerned with the fact that there is such an idea, but it is not concerned with the question whether such an idea is true or false in any other sense. It is psychologically true in as much as it exists. . . . This point of view is the same as that of natural science. . . ."[1]

* * *

The psychological study of every spiritual phenomenon, and particularly that of religious experience, encounters at the outset one fundamental problem which must therefore be discussed first. It is that of *consciousness,* which is inextricably bound up with any spiritual experience. The fact of "being conscious," the attainment of reflection, is what lifts man out of the blind circle of purely biological life. The emergence of consciousness, and with it of a reflective attitude, is the characteristic feature which distinguishes man from the animal. One might even go so far as to define man as the living organism with consciousness. Unfortunately, however, although we have some idea of what consciousness is and how it works, we can say nothing about its origin. The various theories of how it came into being are only deductions from other unproven premises. Thus the extreme materialist would say that the emergence of consciousness is just another variation of biological development, rather in the same line as the step from breathing through gills to breathing through lungs, or from cold blood to warm blood. At the other end of the scale of theories would be that of the religious thinker to whom consciousness is one of the most precious and decisive gifts that God has bestowed on man. If we try, however, to remain on the ground of purely empirical facts, we are bound to admit that we cannot say how and why consciousness originated, any more than we can ascertain anything about how and why life came into existence.

We thus have to take the existence of consciousness for granted as an inexplicable and irreducible phenomenon of human life;

[1]Jung, *Psychology and Religion,* p. 3.

but we can nevertheless try to assess its rôle and define the problems which arise from its emergence. We can say that consciousness has undergone a considerable development from an uncertain and precarious state to a comparatively stable and reliable one, and at the same time that it has, from its very beginning, presented man with an enormous problem, and one that even nowadays is very far from being solved. To be conscious is very far from living in pure bliss; on the contrary, it is just as much a curse as a blessing to the person who experiences it. It is a double-edged weapon, and the experience of its ambiguous character has been expressed in myth after myth. The myth can be regarded as the spontaneous and unreflective formulation of a primal psychological experience of a civilization, and it is for that reason that mythology can teach us so much about the early psychological experiences of mankind. Let us take only two examples: the story of Prometheus and the story of Paradise. The story of Prometheus mirrors all the tremendous dangers that were felt to be inherent in the gift of the light of consciousness; so much so that he who brought this light to mortal man had to commit the tragic crime of violating the laws of the gods, and had to atone for his deed with the eternal wound to the centre of his instinctual life. Even more illuminating is the story of Paradise and the expulsion of man from his blissful state therein. "But of the tree of the knowledge of good and evil, thou shalt not eat of it: for in the day that thou eatest thereof thou shalt surely die"; for man may not be like God, knowing and being conscious. But again man commits the tragic crime of claiming consciousness for himself, and he is driven out of Paradise of preconscious participation in God and out of the divine harmony. What an enormous punishment for an act which meant the beginning of man's history as man! But on the other hand Jewish tradition itself says: "Man was created for the sake of choice," that is, for the sake of the choice between good and evil. To the psychologist the story of Paradise seems rather to express the fear of the enormous burden which consciousness brought to man, together with an equally enormous opportunity. Time and again the psychologist comes across the symbol of Paradise in the dreams and phantasies of his patients. In its regressive aspect it represents the craving for the blissful state in which we were still children without responsibility, when the parents were the gods knowing good and evil, and when one could blindly trust their omniscience without being challenged by the need for one's own discrimination and choice. Nobody likes to be driven out of this paradise of childhood, and mankind in its infancy felt this even more keenly than we, who may be said to have at least found some kind of fragmentary adaptation to the state of consciousness. That is why primitive man needs his cruel—but for that reason all the more impressive—rituals of initiation into manhood, that is into a state of comparative consciousness. They help to erect a kind of wall over which it is not so easy to escape back into "childhood."

There is, however, another reason for the strictness and severity of these initiation rites. It is not only the fear of growing up, fear of consciousness, but equally the fear of losing the still precarious gift of consciousness. This is, in its beginnings, an extremely tender growth which may be uprooted by the slightest opposition. Unconscious emotions may destroy the feared, but nevertheless precious gift on the smallest provocation. Jung mentions in one of his seminars the case of a primitive, a very amiable and gentle creature, who had a little son whom he loved dearly. One day he came back from an unsuccessful fishing expedition. His little son came to meet him, and asked him how much fish he had caught. The man's disappointment flared up into uncontrolled fury, and in his rage he killed his beloved little boy. A second later he was overwhelmed with desperate grief at what he had done. That is how unconscious emotion works where the traces of consciousness are still faint and insecurely established. That is why taboos and collective rituals are so severe and rigid; only a strong fear of the consequences can be relied upon to keep unconscious emotion in check and give consciousness its precarious chance against the vast superiority of its opponent.

I have already mentioned how strong a tendency there is to escape from the yoke of consciousness back into the blissful state of infancy. There are certainly strong reasons for that tendency. The foremost perhaps is that consciousness is equivalent to reflection and discrimination, and therefore inevitably forces us to ask "Why?" and "Wherefore?" That explains, for instance, why people prefer to adhere to so-called collective values and ideas without ever questioning them or enquiring into their validity. We have seen the most striking instances of this in our own time, for every collective situation, such as war, tends to aggravate the preponderance and attraction of collective values. There is nothing that the ordinary human being—and it should be clearly understood that this ordinary human being forms a large part of each one of us—dreads and therefore hates more than the need for discrimination. This is just another way of saying that the knowledge of good and evil is to the collective human mind synonymous with expulsion from Paradise.

This is a point which cannot be too clearly understood and too strongly emphasized: consciousness, and discrimination, is to the ordinary man—the "man in the street" both outside and inside—the arch-enemy. Whenever we can, we try to escape from it and from the yoke which it imposes on us. Yet consciousness, however much we may fear it, is nevertheless our special human characteristic and the power which drives us. One can almost imagine the helpless shock of the poor fish that was driven by some dark but irresistible force out of its beloved water and found itself on that unknown and unloved rough surface called earth, where it had to crawl laboriously along instead of being carried smoothly and gently in the tender surroundings to which it was accustomed. That is the case of man, the animal which woke up out of its unreflective state of being contained in the dark womb of harmonious unconsciousness, and found itself confronted with the problem of existence. A romantic sentimentality has represented primitive man as the prototype of ideal happiness; but how far this is from the truth! Instead of living in a state of undisturbed and unbroken harmony like the animals, primitive man is haunted by psychic fears. His whole life, in so far as it is human life and not mere physiological existence, is one perpetual attempt to adapt to the consequences of consciousness which has descended on him like a demoniacal bird of prey—and the demon has to be propitiated! Taboos and magic are continuous invocations of the still frail power of consciousness against the unconscious, of which man has become aware through the very fact of becoming conscious. Primitive man cannot yet experience these unconscious forces as part of himself. He has to project them—as indeed we project everything that we cannot integrate—into gods, demons, and ghosts. Consciousness is some enigmatic power which has torn him out of his animality. This loss of his preconscious instinctive security may destroy the whole basis of his life unless he can use consciousness, which produced the split, as a protection against the unconscious powers of which he has become aware in his projections. His consciousness is, however, still so young and undeveloped that it does not yet represent a tool to be used without difficulty and hesitation—it has to be invoked with special preparations and rituals. (The medicine-man is the one who, as it were, personifies and carries the collective consciousness, and he therefore knows how to deal with it without being punished by the dark powers of the unconscious—the ghosts and demons.)

As soon as any degree of consciousness is attained, it means that its possessor is no longer indiscriminately contained in the one-ness of life. The one-ness has been split into a great number of different pieces. We can follow this process in the development of the child. At first the child is more or less identical with the parents' psyche—is contained within it. Slowly there emerge out of this primordial ocean of undisturbed uniformity more and more little islands of consciousness, until at last a little individuality begins to take shape. It is an important juncture in his life when a child begins to say "I" instead of calling himself by the name by which he is called by the others. But this little "I," the ego-personality, foreshadows conflict. An ego implies another one, many other ones; and one is no longer just as the others are.

"I" feels opposed to "You"—and the argument of life has been started on its perilous journey. What else are the conflicts of puberty but the attempts of the still delicate ego to assert itself against the other, overpowering egos of the parents or teachers; attempts, as it were, at de-identification with its environment?

Everybody who has had any contact with children knows how closely the awakening of the individuality, of the ego, is linked up with the insatiable and ever-present word "Why?" Matters no longer go without saying, things have to be explained, reasons to be given. Adults never seem to understand, or rather always seem to have forgotten, what an enormous amount of uncertainty this means for the child. What is true of the development of the individual child who suddenly and unexpectedly finds himself confronted with the riddle of the world and of his own existence, is equally true of the development ·of mankind as a whole. It is this fearful bewilderment of the enormous "Why?" and "Wherefore?" that is formulated in the story of the expulsion from Paradise.

But bewilderment asks for an answer. There is one main principle which guides our life, and life altogether. This is the principle of adaptation. Every organism, be it plant, animal or man, has the inherent tendency to adapt to the circumstances with which it finds itself confronted. The tendency to adaptation asserts itself most strongly in every instance where an organism is exposed to new and unknown conditions. Either the organism succeeds in finding its adaptation and so restoring the balance between the forces working on it and its reaction to them, or else it perishes.

Now this, in a purely psychological sense, is the situation in which primitive man must have found himself when consciousness first began to dawn. The fact of being torn out of the preconscious harmony of paradise corresponds, so far as its material effects are concerned, to any other change of circumstances which tears an organism out of a certain set of conditions to which it had found a complete and satisfactory answer. Psychology cannot say anything about the power which caused the

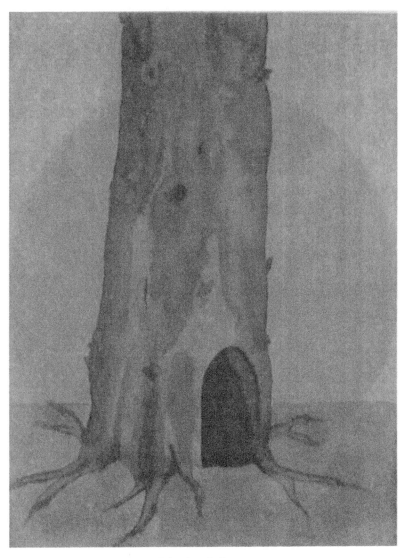

14.   The Dark Door

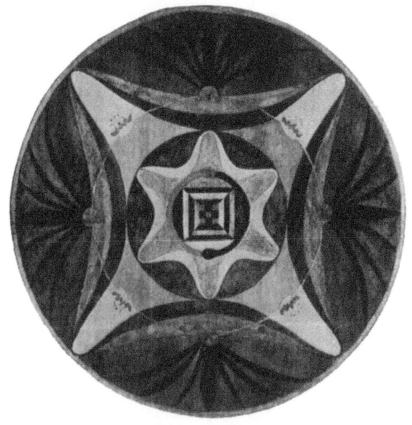

15.   The Dance Pattern

change from the pre-conscious instinctive state to the conscious one. It can only deal with the psychological effects on and the reactions of the organism concerned.

The psychological effect of the emergence of consciousness is the destruction of the balance of correlation between the pre-conscious organism and its merely biological conditioning. In this sense to become conscious means a discrepancy between the organism, which had been adapted to the merely biological pre-conscious state of life, and the new circumstances resulting from consciousness. To become conscious means to discriminate, and discrimination means separation and singling out. Instead of being contained within the biological process of nature, man suddenly found himself at one point beyond this merely biological process owing to the emergence of consciousness, and a new adaptation had to be found.

What man found himself deprived of, through consciousness, was the unquestioning harmony with the world in which he lived. This effect of consciousness is, as far as we can see, unique. Whereas all other biological changes had left the organism concerned still inside the circle of nature, whose only interest seems to be that of self-propagation and the preservation of life, the emergence of consciousness pushed man out of this blind circle. The pre-conscious unity of the biological organism and nature had been torn into two halves: into a subject and an object. It is this state of "dubium," of doubt, of two-ness which, psychologically speaking, is the basis of religion.

The unique situation of man was that he found himself deprived of the pre-conscious harmony and unity with nature. Now an old scholastic saying runs: *"Privatio est causa generationis,"* privation is the cause of generation (creativeness). Aristotle put it in this way: that the beginning of all philosophy is when man begins to wonder. To wonder means to put the two fundamental questions which contain in themselves all others: the question what is the cause and the question what is the purpose, the "Why?" and the "Wherefore?". These two questions with regard to man's position in creation are the real concern of religion.

They are the question about the creating power, and about the meaning of man's life.

It has been said above that the one force which we can observe in every living organism is that of adaptation. In that sense man's attempted answer to these two questions is his adaptation to the enigmatic situation of finding himself charged with consciousness, and thus of being a subject to an object. Every religion is really and truly a system of adaptation to the fact of the emergence of consciousness and the questions which arise from it. If we are to remain on a purely empirical and psychological basis we must say that we know nothing about the so-called objective truth of man's answers. If man in his need for a reply to the question "Why?," that is, to the question what is the *prima causa,* answers: "God is the *prima causa,*" this answer is obviously no evidence in the scientific sense for the existence of God. The same holds good for the answer to the question "Wherefore?". Religion is man's adaptation to this question, and the answer is that there is a definite sense in his existence within the framework of God's creation. Again, we cannot know in a scientific sense whether this answer of ours has any objective validity. To put it in another way: it is beyond the empirical possibilities at our disposal to say whether the meaning that we find in our life is the expression of so-called objective truth.

What we can say, however, is that the answers which man gives in religion are evidence of the most fundamental and crucial *experience* of man, and of the absolute need for this experience. This shows how unsatisfactory and insufficient is the attitude of psychoanalysis (i.e. Freud's school) to the phenomenon of religion and religious phenomena. As has been pointed out above, to psychoanalysis religion is a sublimation of instinctual urges which cannot be realized; in other words it is a substitute for something else. The fact, however, is that religion is not a substitute for something else, but that it stands right at the beginning of man's existence as man, that it is the primal urge of his specific human situation. If we try to explain away the fundamental necessity for religion and its legitimate place in man's psychology, then we try to do away with man as man, and reduce him to a mere fact of biology.

If at this point we try to sum up the result of our psychological analysis, it would be about like this: Man's fate is indissolubly and essentially bound up with and expressed in consciousness, and consciousness is inextricably bound up with and expressed in religion. Religion is man's adaptation to the fact of consciousness; religion is man's reply to his existence as man—and in religion man therefore finds his fullest and most vital expression.

At this point, however, we must carefully guard against a possible misunderstanding. If we say that every religion is a system of adaptation to the fact of man's consciousness and the problems arising from it, it may perhaps sound as if religion, man's answer to his specific situation as man in creation, were a logical and almost arbitrary reply to the challenge. But this is not at all the case, for the answer arises spontaneously in a pre-logical and pre-intellectual, that is in a symbolical, form. Again we may find a parallel to this psychic mechanism in the mind of the child. The child perceives in a pre-logical way—pre-logical, not illogical —that is, in a way in which images seem to emerge out of the primordial ocean of the unconscious. Logical and intellectual man, when he has come up against a problem, answers it through his conscious mind by using his will, which is the energetic expression of his conscious mind. Not so the child or primitive man: to them the answer to any problem arises without a deliberate process out of the depths of their unconscious; and particularly in the case of primitive man it is more than probable that the greater part of his symbols, and thus also of his answers to fundamental problems arises directly from dreams.[1]

Religion is rooted in the unconscious, elemental level in us, and it is from this primordial part of our psyche that the religious images and symbols spring forth. This does not mean, however, that these images and symbols are "primitive" in the sense of outworn, or that they must be discarded as crude approximations, but on the contrary that they are full of symbolical energy,

[1] Cf. Jung, *Contributions to Analytical Psychology*, p. 54f.

i.e. that they express an essence which, although it has not yet arrived at a differentiated formulation, is pregnant with meaning. True religious feeling, just as much as art, is always rooted in this deep level of our psyche. Where it has become logically defined and formulated, we find ourselves in the realm of dogma or in that of philosophy. At this stage it has become differentiated and rationally comprehensible, but it has also lost at least part of its symbolical and numinous quality and with it its power of transformation. This means that in every case where we need an answer which is more than logical and deeper than rational—be it in religion, art, or whatever situation may arise in the process of life—this pre-logical, "primitive" matrix in us, with all its instinctive wisdom, has the power to produce a more meaningful and valid answer than has the conscious mind with its clearer but necessarily more restricted view. For if the unconscious is dimmer and less differentiated, it is also more comprehensive and more full of elemental power.

The fundamental situation which we must understand is the creative polarity between the unconscious and consciousness which has emerged from it. The tension arising out of this polarity sets in motion a process which can best be understood if we compare it to our dreaming. It is not our conscious mind, our ego, our active will, that produces the dream; it arises out of the unconscious. But it is with our conscious mind that we register and observe the emerging images. We know how dim and shadowy our consciousness is in dreams; and this is exactly how we have to understand the state of consciousness in primitive man and in the child. In that sense primitive man and the child live in a continuous state of dreaming.[1] It is quite likely that a similar process goes on in animals, but as there is no consciousness, that is, no partner who could observe what is happening, it is never distinguishable.

What I mean when I speak of man answering the question of

[1]Cf. the remark of a child quoted above ("The Ego and the Cycle of Life," p. 123); "The dream is not in my head, but I am in the dream."

his place in creation, and about his adaptation to this question in religion, is that he is able and indeed bound to give himself up to observing this inner stream and urge of emerging images. Primitive man and the child are enclosed "within their dream," that is within the all-enveloping primeval womb of life, with just enough light to observe dimly what is happening. It is the polarity between the night of the primeval womb and the light of consciousness that has been born out of it, which produces the human drama.[1] The tragic temptation arising from this situation is to give more and more importance to the conscious mind until we deceive ourselves into believing that it is the conscious mind which is the creative power. This temptation forms the specific tragic conflict of the human drama. This problem will be dealt with later.

It has been mentioned before that from the point of view of psychology we cannot say anything about the objective existence of God. But what was said just now about the images emerging out of the unconscious shows the problem in a new light and makes it possible to place it in its proper perspective. If it is not man's deliberate will which produces the answers to his question—answers which in that case might even be arbitrary attempts at self-deception—where then do they come from? Again it must be emphasized that as psychologists we have to avoid any metaphysical or religious explanations. All we can say at this point is that we do not know what power makes the answers emerge from the dark realm of pure images. We can however ascertain certain facts about the dynamic process of this creation of images.

One such fact is that mankind, at every stage in its development and in vastly different circumstances, has always produced images of the creative power, the Deity, which although different in detail show a surprising and convincing conformity in principle. This characteristic they have in common with other ele-

---

[1] Cf. Appendix (p. 215), in which an example is given showing how this process has been formulated in mystical experience.

mental images of a numinous character, such as the image of the "Great Mother" or of the "night journey under the sea." From the fact that man does not deliberately invent such images, we may assume that they arise out of a common structure of the human psyche. In as far as they are not conscious formulations but rather images that force themselves on man's conscious realization, we can say that they arise out of man's unconscious. Jung has called this common structure of the human psyche the *collective,* or *supra-personal,* unconscious, and the images emerging from it he has termed the *archetypes.* The archetypes, then, are "primordial figures of the unconscious."[1] In as far as they belong to the layer of the collective *unconscious,* they are psychic contents that have not yet been subjected to conscious treatment, and so represent "an immediate, psychic actuality."[2]

It has been said above that we can understand the psychological process, just as we can any biological process, from the point of view of adaptation. With the idea of the archetypes as an immediate psychic actuality in mind, we can now understand how the conscious and the unconscious psyche work together to produce the specific human adaptation. The conscious mind is separated from its pre-conscious matrix, and thus an inner tension arises which acts as a stimulus to find its solution. This stimulus is answered by the unconscious which, as it were, sends up an image as a response to the unsatisfactory situation of inner tension. This response is not a deliberate attempt of the conscious mind, but a reaction of the unconscious, and can therefore be regarded as an instinctive reaction. Just as instincts are typical ways of action and reaction, so too are the archetypes. They are "a living system of reactions and aptitudes determining the individual—that is conscious—life."[3] Just as instincts are unconscious, biologically necessary responses to certain stimuli, so are the archetypes unconscious, psychologically necessary responses to certain other stimuli. Kant has called the instincts "internal

[1] Jung, *The Integration of the Personality,* p. 23.
[2] Ibid., p. 54.
[3] Jung, *Contributions to Analytical Psychology,* p. 117.

necessities," and equally the archetypes are an internal necessity of the human psyche. They are, as it were, "organs of the psyche."[1]

The archetypes are, of course, not closely circumscribed ideas which are reproduced under the impact of the stimulus, but rather unconscious inherited predispositions to certain reactions. Jung has compared the archetypes to the axial system of a crystal. He says: "The form of these archetypes is perhaps comparable to the axial system of a crystal which predetermines as it were the crystalline formation in the saturated solution, without itself possessing a material existence. This existence first manifests itself in the way the ions and then the molecules arrange themselves. . . . The axial system determines, accordingly, merely the stereometric structure, not, however, the concrete form of the individual crystal . . . and just so the archetype possesses . . . an invariable core of meaning that determines its manner of appearing always only in principle, never concretely."[2] In this sense the archetypes are pre-existent and immanent as a potential axial system. The images are existent *in potentia* in the collective unconscious, and it is the impact of human consciousness that changes the potential image into the actual one, that is into the experience of the archetype. The archetypes are therefore "an eternal presence,"[3] but whether they are ever realized depends on whether the individual becomes aware of them or not.

The most powerful archetypal experience of man is that of the "Deity." As a matter of fact, from the standpoint of psychology this statement has to be reversed, and we have to say that man has called his most powerful experience: "God." It is the experience of a supra-individual centre of existence, of a power that gives and takes life, of a point from which life springs and towards which it aims, and in which the meaning and purpose of creation and man's place in it seem to become apparent. In this

[1]Jung, *Das Göttliche Kind*, Pantheon, Amsterdam, Leipzig, 1940, p. 47.
[2]Jung, *Die psychologischen Aspekte des Mutterarchetypus*. In: Eranos Jahr-Buch, 1938, Zürich, 1939, p. 410.
[3]Jung, *The Integration of the Personality*, p. 200.

archetypal experience of the "Deity" the polarity between the unconscious and the conscious psyche finds its synthesis, and the tension is resolved in a complete union of the opposites. It is an immediate and direct experience of an absolutely convincing character, and one that carries with it a feeling of self-evidence. It is not *made* by man but *happens* to him out of the depth of his psychic existence. In other words, it is a spontaneous occurrence whose psychic reality cannot be denied.

Jung has termed this psychic fact the "self," in order to avoid any dogmatic limitation and because an indefinite term best expresses the indefinable character of this experience. Every experience of the Deity, whether it be formulated as Jahwe, Christ, Buddha or in any other way, thus represents, psychologically speaking, the experience of the self as the psychic totality and the union of the opposites—the *"coincidentia oppositorum."* This does not contain any statement about the existence or non-existence of God. Jung has pointed out that what is meant by the word "archetype" is the "type in the psyche," which comes from τυπός, i.e. imprint or impression, and that therefore "the very word 'archetype' postulates something which imprints."[1] Psychology, however, cannot say "what, in the last instance, the archetype is derived from, any more than we know the origin of the psyche."[2] Thus "the religious standpoint naturally places the emphasis on that which makes the imprint; *the scientific standpoint, on the other* hand, *regards it as a* symbol of a content which is unknown to it and beyond its grasp."[3] Regarded from the psychological standpoint the self can thus be formulated as the experience of the "God within us," whereas to religion the self would be a manifestation of "God in Himself."

This fact of the existence is the psyche of an archetype which man has termed "God" and its actualization through the impact of the conscious mind takes us to the end of our empirical and

[1] Jung, *Psychologie und Alchemie*, p. 28.
[2] Ibid.
[3] Ibid., p. 33.

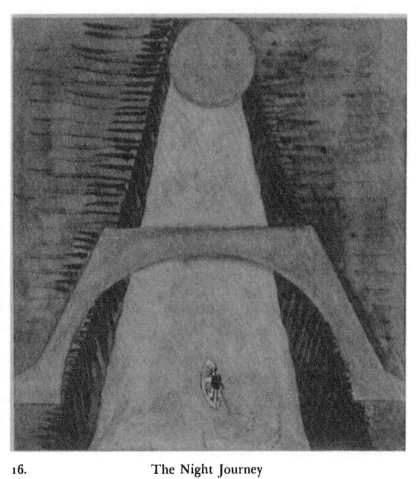

16.   The Night Journey

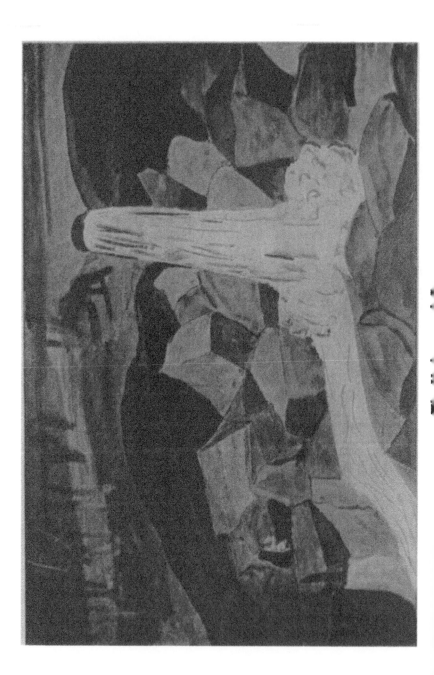

psychological statements. All that we can say, strictly speaking, is that religion is a fundamental activity of the human mind, and that there exists an archetypal image of the Deity deeply and indestructibly engraved in our psyche. Psychology cannot prove or disprove the existence of God; what it can prove, however, is the existence of an archetypal image of God, the "self." Here, then, psychology and religion both part and meet, facing each other from different sides of the frontier. All that psychology can legitimately do is to look across and to accept the possibility that the "God within us" corresponds to a transcendental reality.

Goethe has expressed this thought in his beautiful verses:

> "Wär nicht das Auge sonnenhaft,
> Die Sonne könnt' es nie erblicken;
> Läg nicht in uns des Gottes eigne Kraft,
> Wie könnt'uns Göttliches entzücken?"[1]

II

In the course of the preceding discussion of the part played by consciousness in the phenomenon of religion, a particular problem has become visible. It is that of the polarity between consciousness and the unconscious matrix from which it springs. This polarity develops only too easily into an open conflict when the unconscious and the conscious psyche become alienated from one another and split asunder.

This conflict is inherent in the nature both of the unconscious and of the conscious psyche. Both have their constructive and their destructive side, and if the latter gains the upper hand, the split becomes inevitable. In its creative aspect the unconscious is the container of all instincts, and from that source everything creative flows. As "the totality of all archetypes," it is "the deposit of all human experience back to its most remote be-

[1] "If the eye were not of sun-like nature, it could never see the sun; if the power of the Deity itself did not lie within us, how could we take delight in the Divine?"

ginnings."[1] It is prior to the conscious mind, it is its mother and its eternal nourishment. At the same time the unconscious needs this its child in order to be realized; without the reflecting conscious mind there would be no consciousness of the unconscious either. This is the essential difference between man and animal. Although the unconscious and the conscious mind need each other—the conscious mind being the condition of realization of the unconscious, while the unconscious is the constantly creative matrix of the conscious mind—they may turn against each other and in so doing reveal their destructive aspects. The conscious mind may forget its source and the condition of its life—which is the constant relatedness to the unconscious as the container of the instincts and of the supra-individual experience—and may thus cut itself loose from its own nourishing roots. The unconscious on the other hand, through its very superiority and through its impersonal nature, may turn against its child and destroy it. In this case the mother has revealed her devouring aspect, unconcerned about the individual, interested only in the blind circle of creation as such. The conscious mind, on the other hand, may become so fascinated by the power of its mother that it sacrifices its *raison d'être,* its faculty of reflection and discrimination, and is sucked back into the dark womb of the unconscious night. Only a mutual relationship between the two in which each partner fulfils its innate destiny can reveal the creative meaning of both. This problem will now be discussed in some of its implications.

It has been said above that consciousness is the specifically human achievement, and it has been shown how the existence of man is fundamentally and indissolubly bound up with and expressed in the fact of becoming conscious. Is it surprising, then, that man should feel that this specific gift of his is the only thing that matters? Man behaves like the child who is beginning for the first time to feel his own individual powers and rejects any help and advice from the superior knowledge of his parents. Jung has said: "Our consciousness, being still young

[1]Jung, *Contributions to Analytical Psychology,* p. 116.

and frail, has a tendency to make little of the unconscious. This is understandable enough, for a young boy should not be too deeply impressed by the majesty of his parents if he wants to accomplish something in his own right and way."[1] It is understandable enough if we bear in mind what an enormous effort and risk it means to man to become conscious. The constant fear of primitive man is that he may lose this precarious dim light of first awareness; and how else could such a delicate light be protected from extinction but by every effort and attention being concentrated upon it? That is why man is fascinated by this new gift and acquirement which, strictly speaking, was thrust upon him.

Ever since its first beginnings, human history has been the history of a constant development and differentiation of consciousness. In the early stages man was still very close to the unconscious matrix, the great creative darkness from which his consciousness had sprung; but with ever increasing distance from the first pangs of birth, consciousness forgot its origin and tended to become more and more autocratic. That this process of hypertrophic over-development of the conscious ego must be inherent in the relationship between the conscious and the unconscious psyche, and how early a conflict appeared, is clearly indicated by such a story as that of the Tower of Babel. And we find the same hypertrophic development of the conscious mind illustrated in Plato's story of how the sexes became separated and the wholeness of man cut into two halves. It was a punishment of the gods because man had over-reached himself, and felt like one of them, "knowing good and evil."[2] With the growth of consciousness this conflict became more and more critical.

The hypertrophic development of the conscious mind is inherent in its very nature. To be conscious means to discriminate, and discrimination means concentration on some few contents which by this very process of concentration attain a new light of clarity. The conscious mind works by excluding

[1] Jung, *The Integration of the Personality*, p. 12.
[2] Cf. "Consciousness and Cure," p. 139.

all contents on which it is not focused, and is thus always bound to be more or less one-sided. The more the conscious mind, and its representative the ego, become differentiated, the more easily may they become instruments for using the power of the will in an arbitrary way. Primitive man cannot use his budding conscious mind as a willing tool. If he wants to do something, his will has first to be stimulated by all kinds of initiation rites, so-called *rites d'entrée,* which help to make the unconscious energy flow towards the conscious purpose. If primitive man wants, for example, to go to war, or on a hunting expedition, he cannot simply say "I shall go," but has first, in the war-dance or similar rituals, to rouse his dim and dormant will to the level of his intended action. It is obvious how much superior civilized man's conscious and differentiated will is, since it provides him with an adequate tool to execute his intentions. Primitive man could never rouse his will beyond intentions and desires which express his natural instincts; but that is exactly what civilized man can and does do. Will, the instrument of the conscious mind, is thus at the same time his great potentiality and his equally great danger. It is a potentiality because it represents an enormous source of human freedom and independence, and a danger because it is a constant cause of one-sidedness, lack of relatedness, and loss of the instinctive roots.[1]

The problem, then, has always been how to make use of the constructive power of the conscious mind without turning it against its indispensable partner, the unconscious, in which it is rooted. Man soon became aware of the danger inherent in the conscious mind, namely that it might cut itself off from its life-giving roots; and he took his precautions against this danger. He tried to remind himself constantly of the fact that a power greater than his ego, i.e. a "non-ego," dwelt behind his conscious activity. A formula such as the *"Deo volente,"* "God willing," which he added to his planning and scheming was a pregnant warning to himself that whatever man may try to do by an act of his free will, he has to remember that after all some other factor which

[1] Cf. Jung, *Das Göttliche Kind,* p. 100ff.

is not of his own making has a say in his decision. Thus this formula was meant as a constant reminder as well as a kind of propitiatory gesture to the unknown and unaccountable power behind our will; it is a kind of magic charm with which to avert its wrath, which might be aroused by man's autocratic behaviour.

This problem has a long history. I have tried to show how religion is not an act of conscious deliberation and intellectual discrimination but how it grows quite spontaneously out of the pre-conscious depths of the human psyche. It is the numinous images of the collective unconscious, the archetypes, which first become visible to and through man's consciousness. Foremost among them is the archetype of the Deity in which man perceives the power, or the powers, which control and direct his life and destiny. Religious practice is—to use Jung's words—the "careful consideration and observation of certain dynamic factors, understood to be powers,"[1] whether they be called spirits, demons, gods, ideas, or whatever else. Primitive man has still not lost the knowledge that these powers are beyond the reach of his will, but that they control the human subject, which is not their creator but rather their victim. In this sense the "numinosum," as Rudolf Otto has called this power, "is an involuntary condition of the subject."[2] All that man can do is to observe the miraculous ways of this numinosum and thus learn to make use of them, or rather to adapt to them, at least up to a point. This is the original idea behind all religious and ritualistic performances. Religious practice aims at constantly linking man up again with this power or powers, and thus keeping alive the connection between man's conscious mind and its source.

The necessity for doing this explains why so many primitive tribes have perished under the impact of the white man. The mythology of a tribe is its living and organically growing religion; it is its particular system of archetypes and constellation of guiding powers. The superior intellect of the white man destroys this pattern of living religion, so that the tribe loses its

[1]Jung, *Psychology and Religion*, p. 3.
[2]Ibid., p. 4.

soul, and with it its morale and cohesion. For the myth of a tribe, and indeed every myth, is not a conscious and deliberate invention, but a genuine revelation of the supra-personal and pre-conscious psyche, of the collective unconscious. Religion in its beginning is a coherent and organic pattern of myths, and this pattern represents a dynamic and living relatedness to the eternal images in the unconscious. Where this relation is disturbed, the whole organism withers away.

What is true of primitive man is equally true of modern man. Our creative attitude, the childlike originality of our experience of the "numinosum," is in constant danger of being disturbed and destroyed by a more highly differentiated but fatally one-sided and unrooted will. The results are only too obvious if we look at the statistics of suicides and psychoneuroses, not to mention the more infernal effects of modern man's loss of instinctive relatedness.

Yet we cannot escape our fate and cast off the yoke of consciousness. To become conscious is the prerogative of man, and in the process of reflection he steps out of the blind circle of nature. This means that it is equally dangerous to man to cling to the merely instinctive side of his existence. The conscious mind and the will always want to progress. As a result they are in danger of cutting man off from his natural roots, and pushing him into abstract and unnatural ideas. This, however, is the risk in all development, and if it were not accepted there would be no progress and no future. On the opposite side there stands the ideal of relatedness to the instincts and of loyalty to the roots. Though this idea keeps man sane and stable, it may on the other hand also condemn him to inertia and a superstitious conservatism. The truth, as always, seems to lie neither on the one side nor on the other, but in a synthesis of the two. Jung once half jokingly remarked: "My psychology is not a psychology of the either-or, but a psychology of the either-and-or." If man seems to be suspended in mid-air between the two poles of the conscious ego and his active will on the one hand and the supra-personal and timeless unconscious on the other. if in this bed of Procrustes he finds himself either too large or too small—is it possible to find an answer that comprises the either and the or?

It is necessary to realize that this is not merely an isolated problem, but really the main problem of our time. In every sphere of life we seem to be confronted with this same problem of being torn between the timeless unchanging past with all its attraction of stability and security and its danger of sterility and petrifaction, and the constantly moving future with its chance of development and growth and its danger of isolation from the instinctive roots and its lack of coherence. This unconscious conflict between the fundamental pair of opposites is perceptible, for instance, behind the conflict between political conservatism and communism. Both these political attitudes can be understood as instances of the archetypal conflict between the past and the future. This conflict is so much part and parcel of our inner life that we are bound to project our own inner problems into it, and thus to lose all detachment and objectivity. And what is true of politics is true of every department of life in which human activity can express itself. Everywhere there seems to be conflict between the past and the future, and everywhere it calls for conscious decisions and new realizations.

Is it surprising, then, that we should be faced with this same problem in religion which, after all, in its concern for the question of the inner meaning of our life, plays such a crucial part? In the field of religion the problem is that of the relation between the collective religious ritual and the individual religious experience. In a certain sense this problem could be described as that of the relationship—and often conflict—between the priest and the prophet. It is not my task to go into the historical aspect of the matter, and I shall confine myself to the psychological significance of this inner tension in man's religious experience.

Let us, therefore, first consider what are the implications of the two attitudes or experiences. It is the concern of religion to find an answer to the question of the meaning and significance of our life. The answer to this question is no arbitrary intellectual process, but arises spontaneously out of the depths of the human psyche. It is the primal experience of the "numinosum," presenting itself with all the terrific impact of its supraindividual power. Rudolf Otto has described this aspect of the numinosum as the "tremendum" or the "fascinans."[1] It is the experience of the "living God." We have a great many descriptions of the overwhelming force of this experience, from the oldest times to the experiences of modern mystics. It is the power which overwhelms man, tears him with irresistible force away from his accustomed way of life, a hard and uncompromising hand which cannot be averted, the voice from which there is no escape, the storm that seizes and drives man and shakes him like the leaves of the aspen, the fire that burns and purifies him until at last all that remains of him is the unassailable and terrifying mouth of God. "Mine heart within me is broken; all my bones shake; I am like a drunken man, and like a man whom wine has overcome, because of the Lord, and because of the words of His holiness," says Jeremiah.

What happens, psychologically speaking, is that the individual is overcome by the power of the archetype of the Deity, that he is face to face, without a protecting veil, with the blinding light of the symbol of the centre of life. But this centre of life is also the very centre of death to the one who is not fully prepared for it, as Korah and his followers as well as the Philistines had to find out. Every original encounter with that force which man has termed "God," with the archetype of the fateful power that gives and takes life, means potential death. Every return from this crucial experience is to be reborn from the depths of utter extinction. There are two stories of two Hasidic rabbis[2] which illustrate this point beautifully. This is the first:

---

[1] Cf. Rudolf Otto, *Das Heilige*, Beck, Munich, 1917, particularly the two chapters "Mysterium tremendum" and "Das Fascinans." (Translated by John W. Harvey under the title *The Idea of the Holy*, Oxford University Press, 1923.)

[2] The Hasidim were a mystical sect in Judaism, founded by Rabbi Israel Baal-Shem-Tov in the eighteenth century. The two stories are taken from Martin Buber: *Die Chassidischen Bücher*, Hegner, Hellerau, 1928, pp. 573, 574.

"Somebody asked Rabbi Salaman of Karlin to come and see him the following day. The Rabbi answered: 'How can you ask me for a promise? To-night I have to pray and to say the "Hear, O Israel"[1] and my soul will go to the edge of life. Then there will be the darkness of sleep; and in the morning I shall say the great morning-prayer which is a going through all worlds, and finally I shall have to fall down on my face, and my soul will bend itself over the edge of life. Perhaps I shall not die this time, but how shall I promise to do anything after my prayer?' " And the other story: "Before he went to say his prayers Rabbi Uri used each morning to put his house in order and take leave from his wife and children."

That is why the mystics talk about the "emptiness" or "nothingness" as the core of their experience. It is the surrender and the extinction of the individual ego as nearly as it can be without complete and final extinction; and how often may it have been beyond return? "For who is there of all flesh, that hath heard the voice of the living God speaking out of the midst of the fire, as we have, and lived?" This is also the story of many an artist—and here true art and religious experience speak of the same dynamic force—who gave himself up to the fascination of the primordial images and was caught by their fateful power that burst the integrity of his individuality.

Nowhere, however, is man so near the "fire" that means either death or rebirth as in his religious experience. "It is a fearful thing to fall into the hands of the living God"—and "Our God is a consuming fire" says Paul in the Epistle to the Hebrews. It is the most undiluted experience of the numinosum—of the non-ego—that man can have, in which its vast superiority over the ego becomes obvious. Is it to be wondered at that man, whose deepest craving is for the revelation of this power, is at the same time terrified lest it should devour him? That is the reason why men from the very beginning have built protective walls and tried to canalize the terrifying energy of the original experience. This is the function of the ritual.

[1]The "Hear, O Israel" is the central profession of faith of the Jewish religion.

It is obvious that before the ritual there must have been the original, unritualized experience of the numinosum. This was the experience of the individual ego as it was confronted with the power of the supra-personal image. The impact was such that man felt that this power had to be propitiated lest it should destroy him. In order to be approached the Infinite had to be described in symbols, and the system of these finally formed the accepted creed. The symbol thus acts as a "transformer of energy" through which the original energy of the unconscious becomes available to the conscious mind.

There are obviously good and sound reasons for such a body of rituals and symbols because the original unlimited experience of the archetype of the Deity creates a tremendous danger for the coherence of the personality. For the conscious mind is not and cannot at all times be strong enough to act as an equal partner to the numinous power arising out of the unconscious. This danger exists for collective society in which only a few individuals, called medicine-men, priests, prophets, saints and so on, are integrated enough to withstand and assimilate the impact of the numinosum; and it exists equally for the individual, who can act in this integrated way only in relatively short moments of intense concentration. If the ritual acts as a protection, it likewise acts as an instrument. For through its symbolical formulations the less integrated individual is able to approach the numinosum right up to the border of the last experience, and thus to participate to a greater or lesser degree, according to his capacity, in the original experience.

This is the creative function of a ritual, and it is therefore a necessity to the collective personality, both inner and outer. In the act of the ritual, which reproduces the original numinous experience of the most integrated individuals, the ego is constantly reminded of the existence of, and brought into contact with, the non-ego, the supra-personal and preconscious power as it manifests itself to the conscious mind in the archetypal images. To use Jung's words: "In the ritual act man places himself at the disposal of an autonomous 'Eternal,' i.e. of a cause existing beyond all the categories of the conscious mind."[1]

That is why every true ritual legitimately claims to be based on revelation. "Revelation," psychologically speaking, is always the emergence of the numinous non-ego in the form of archetypal images in the conscious mind, and in so far as these archetypal images are "eternal," they contain a "truth" and wisdom that infinitely transcends the knowledge of the ego. Thus these images have the character of "revelation," i.e. of facts, otherwise unknowable, offered to the realization of the ego. Such rituals as those of the Christian Easter or the Jewish Day of Atonement are channels through which facts which belong to the eternal laws of the human psyche are meant to be re-lived in a process of directed meditation, "as if a window were opened or a door pushed open towards the non-spatial or the non-temporal."[2] Inside the circle of the ritual lies the guarantee of the possible relation to and connection with the experience of the Deity, if the conscious mind can make it yield its original meaning. In this sense ritual is the mediator between the supra-individual non-ego and the individual ego.

Compared with the collective, supra-individual unconscious, the conscious mind is a very ephemeral affair. Each individual experience, compared with the unconscious, is like a passing bubble on the surface of the ocean. The conscious mind is constantly changing and moving; the unconscious on the other hand is without time, is everlasting. It is a general belief among primitives—and we also find distinct traces of it in the Bible—that man was originally immortal, and that he lost his immortality merely by accident or by mistake. The accident or mistake is nothing but the fact of the emergence of consciousness. To become conscious does indeed make man "mortal," and this idea is also expressed in the story of Paradise and the first sin. That is why the philosopher Proclus said: "Where there is creation, there is time."

---

[1]Jung, *Das Wandlungssymbol in der Messe*. In: Eranos Jahr-Buch, 1940–41, Zürich, 1942, p. 124.

[2]Ibid., p. 82.

The unconscious, on the other hand, is timeless eternity and immortal duration. It is obvious that the short-lived conscious ego may be liable to tragic mistakes and misjudgments. Has this ephemeral, passing ego any right to set itself against the eternal timelessness of the pre-conscious matrix? Is the longing for individual experience more than a childish desire to turn its own unimportance into the centre of a world which laughs at its futility and shakes it off with a condescending or impatient gesture?

But this question is in itself a fallacy. For the unconscious only has substance to man through its realization by his conscious mind. The unconscious and the conscious psyche form two poles each of which is indispensable to the other. If the unconscious is a vastly superior and truly creative power, the individual ego with its consciousness is the instrument through which this creative power expresses itself, and without which it could never be actualized in human terms. Psychologically speaking, the realizing subject as expressed in individual consciousness is the absolutely indispensable counterpart to the eternity of creation as expressed in the unconscious. Without this subject, creation would not exist as far as man is concerned.[1] The same holds good for the relation between the archetypal experience as expressed in ritual, and the individual experience.

To use the pattern of dialectical development as an illustration, the collective unconscious would be the thesis, and the conscious mind the antithesis. In every sense the conscious mind represents the opposite pole to the unconscious. The unconscious is timeless and static; the conscious mind is in time, and it is in dynamic movement. The unconscious is passive, while the conscious mind is active. It wants to separate, to discriminate, whereas the unconscious rests in the complete one-ness of all life. The unconscious is collective in its state of pre-differentiation;

[1] James Sully, in his *Studies of Childhood* (London, 1895), reports this interesting case: "A little boy of five who was rather given to saying 'clever' things, was once asked by a visitor, who thought to rebuke what he took to be his conceit: 'Why, M., however did the world go round before you came into it?' M. at once replied: 'Why, it *didn't* go round. It only began five years ago.'" (l.c. p. 118.)

the conscious mind constantly tends to differentiate. This is indeed the inner law of the conscious mind; without its separation from the matrix, its differentiation and individualization, the indispensable other pole of existence would be lacking. The conscious mind, as it were, actualizes the very fact of the unconscious, for the latter would be meaningless without the realizing ego. In this sense to become conscious is "part of the divine process of life, or, in other words, God becomes manifest in the human act of reflection."[1]

In a way the polarity between the unconscious and the conscious mind poses the old metaphysical problem of why God should have created the world, since He is perfect in Himself and without need of anything outside His own existence. It is a problem that cannot be answered logically. Following the line of the metaphysical argument we might, however, say that man must have been in immanent quality of the divine personality without which He and His creation would have been incomplete. Man was God's immanent partner in creation—the opposite pole through which God became a realized and conscious fact.

Psychologically speaking, this problem is that of the relationship between the self and the ego. What happens in consciousness, of which man is the bearer, can be understood as "a spontaneous manifestation of the self that existed for ever . . ." and "the revelation of an existence which is pre-existent with regard to the ego, and even its father or creator and its totality."[2] This explains why man, in spite of his fear of consciousness, cannot escape the urge to become conscious. Although consciousness means the sacrifice of the eternal unity and harmony with the self, it is this very self which asks for the sacrifice by sacrificing its own transcendence. In consciousness the self has admitted the factor of time and mortality in order to become an actual individual event.

To express the psychological situation in a simile, we might say that the "first sin" is thus not only a failure of the first man

[1]Jung, *Zur Psychologie der Trinitätsidee*, p. 47.
[2]Jung, *Das Wandlungssymbol in der Messe*, p. 144.

but at the same time an admission of God's need for completion through man's consciousness—the self needs the ego in order to become manifest. Whereas the relationship between God and man was originally meant to be one of eternal harmony, the first sin revealed an inexplicable flaw in God's creation, and if we may say so, an inexplicable imperfection in the divine personality. This divine imperfection became personified in the person of the Devil. The Devil is, as it were, God's dissatisfaction with Himself, a projection of His own doubt.[1] This is the Lucifer-aspect of the Devil; he acts as a constant reminder of the flaw in creation, and thus as a constant urge towards conscious realization and thereby towards greater perfection. This rôle is beautifully illustrated by the function of the Devil in the Book of Job. It is God's own doubt of the correctness of His own creation which drives Him to the experiment with Job in which this creation of His has to justify itself. In this sense Lucifer plays a similar part to that of the Platonic Eros, who is the great instigator of unrest, the urge towards completeness, the "striving for wholeness."

Just as Eros has its destructive aspect, the obsession with merely sensual lust, so Satan is the destructive aspect of the Devil. Satan means literally "the one who interferes," "who prevents." This is not Lucifer who makes things happen because he is the necessary expression of the world's imperfection; he is the Devil who has cut himself loose from God. This is exactly the situation of the conscious mind when it has cut its links with the unconscious. Where the conscious mind becomes hypertrophic, where it tries to assume the sole direction and responsibility, it is bound in the long run to act as "Satan," interfering and preventing instead of urging and stimulating.

On the other hand, a corresponding danger is inherent in ritual. Ritual is, as has been said before, the collectivized formulation of the original individual experience of the supra-individ-

---

[1] In a Persian story the origin of Ahriman—the principle of evil—is explained by a doubting thought of Ahuramazda, the good principle. (Quoted from Jung, *Zur Psychologie der Trinitätsidee*, p. 56.)

ual power. It is an attempt to "regularize" the experience of the numinosum; to make it approachable to every man according to his capacity. Although the original meaning of the ritual is thus that of mediation, of a channel between the supra-individual power—the non-ego—and the individual conscious mind—the ego—there is a danger that the ritual may become more and more formalized. Every ritual tends to build more and more fences round the numinosum, thus in the end suffocating what it was meant to guard. Instead of being an instrument of constant renewal, ritual may become a "protection" against the energy of the immediate experience to such an extent that the immediate experience is lost behind the protective walls. Instead of being a legitimate protection against disintegration through the immediate experience of the "living God," and at the same time a guarantee of participation in that experience, it turns into a weapon against individual experience. The ritual inevitably becomes a function of the collectivity, and every collectivity in the end feels itself menaced by the novelty and unpredictability of the individual experience.[1]

No collectivity is more conservative than primitive society, because primitive man is so extremely afraid of losing his precariously established and still fragmentary ego in the encounter with the superior force of the unconscious images. The new and unknown experience may also open the door to new and unknown dangers, and with the ego and the will still so undeveloped, they may be completely overrun by these forces. Primitive man and the primitive part in each one of us have the *horror novi*, the horror of change, and act accordingly. This is the point at which the ritual may become sterile. It loses its original significance as a mediator between ego and non-ego, and becomes instead an instrument of denial and rejection of the numinous as a living influence in the life of the individual.[2]

[1] A classical representation of this conflict has been given by Dostoievski in the story of the encounter between the Grand Inquisitor and Christ in his *The Brothers Karamazov*.

[2] It has to be emphasized that this represents only the manifestation of the danger inherent in the ritual, but is certainly not the *necessary* development.

This conflict becomes more and more apparent with the growth of the conscious mind. The ego, the representative of the conscious mind, that is still so small and precarious in primitive man, has considerably enlarged its hold and increased its integrity in the course of its development. In this process the ego has become more and more alienated from the living force of the non-ego. Either the non-ego is shut away in a formalized and devitalized ritual to which no genuine function is attributed, or the ego rejects it completely and believes in its own omnipotence. In the first case the ritual no longer acts as an instrument of actualization of the numinous, as "a window towards the Eternal," but represents merely a kind of propitiatory magic through which the non-ego is kept at a distance. In the second case the energy gained by the development of the ego is not used to create a stronger and more continuous conscious realization of the relationship between the ego and the non-ego (thus a process of mutual fertilization), but for an autocratic rule of the powers of the will. Because the revelation of the supra-individual power through the archetypal images, as it is formulated in the ritual, needs consciousness as a counterpole to become manifest and actual, the conscious mind may deceive itself into believing that it is the *maker* of the revelation and begin to ascribe to itself divine powers of creation. The dependence of the ego upon the sources of the non-ego is overlooked, and the result is a growing loss of instinctive relatedness and of knowledge of the natural limitations and conditions of the ego.

Thus the two poles of the ego and the non-ego, which are dependent upon mutual co-operation for productive work, have been torn asunder and turned against one another. This conflict is at the bottom of our cultural crisis, which has assumed such terrible proportions. But just as the individual neurosis, in spite of its unpleasant and even disastrous effects, is nevertheless the last attempt of the psyche to force a new and better

---

There are, of course, always a great number of individuals who have not lost the original meaning of the ritual. They are the true believers in every creed. The petrifaction of the ritual is, however, sufficiently apparent as an important development and one which has a negative influence on its rôle in religious practice.

adaptation on the individual, so our cultural neurosis may be regarded as having the same quality. A new sense of urgency has grown up among many people and is undoubtedly the first sign of an attempt at a new synthesis.

Any solution of the conflict which may be reached will necessarily be different according to whether the individual still feels that his deepest urges are expressed in some established creed, and thus feels himself satisfactorily contained within the symbolism and ritual of that creed, or whether, as is the case with only too many modern people, no creed and no established ritual seems to express his inner need. Nevertheless, both attempts at a synthesis have in common the rediscovered realization of the interdependence of the eternal supra-individual images and the individual conscious mind.

From this position a new vitalization of the ritual becomes possible. Where ritual has come to be misunderstood as a fixed code of ceremonial behaviour, as a kind of collective guarantee of being on the "right side," individual consciousness has been surrendered for the sake of conforming to the general standard. But although a danger of collective encrustation is inherent in ritual, it exists only when ritual has degenerated. To the individual who approaches the ritual action with an inner preparedness to encounter the numinosum, the original archetypal experience of the Deity and its manifestations become significant again. With such an attitude the supra-individual, eternal images are approached by the ego that maintains its individual dignity, that knows of its rôle as the counterpole to the supra-individual. In such an approach the connection between the numinous symbols of the ritual and the individual consciousness has been re-created. Quite apart from all those cases which still rest safely in their relatedness to a ritual and dogma, or those cases which rediscover such a relatedness in the normal process of life, psychologists know of plenty of cases of people who come for analytical treatment, and in its course rediscover their genuine allegiance to a creed. For them the obvious solution is to follow their inner experience and to accept what they believed they had lost.

What, however, of all the other ones—and their number is considerable—who suffer because they feel their spiritual isolation and loneliness, and who would wish for nothing better than to find their way back into an established creed, but to whom this way remains closed? Are they lost to the "mysterium" behind the ritual and thus to "salvation"?

How this question is to be answered depends upon one's point of view with regard to the rôle of the established creed; and psychology is not called upon to judge what answer is right, but merely to describe what happens. The fact is that to many people the access to established creeds and rituals is blocked for some reason or other. Some feel that these creeds, during their long development, have reached such a high degree of differentiation that the natural unconscious energy has evaporated out of their ritual.[1] They feel that to many faithful believers dogma and ritual have accumulated such power that the "external object of worship . . . precisely through the veneration of its object, prevents the soul from being affected in its depths. . . . The divine mediator remains as an image outside, but the man remains fragmentary and his deepest nature is not touched."[2] To others it is repugnant or simply impossible to accept a solution that is given from outside and presented as collectively obligatory. Many feel a discrepancy between the dogmas and contents of an accepted creed and the manner in which its obligations and implications are evaded in actual life. For these or other reasons they cannot find a way back to the established symbols and creeds; and nevertheless—they may have intense religious experience in the sense of feeling some power

---

[1] This feeling also explains why so many people, in the search for the meaning of their lives, are fascinated by so-called esoteric doctrines, whether they be formulated as theosophy, yoga, occultism or in other ways. They seem to contain "numinous" value simply through the fact that our intellect has not yet "spoiled" them. Being so "unknown"—so much the "wholly other"—they represent a more suitable object for the projection of unconscious energies than the known and intellectualized symbols of our own civilization. Just this fact, however, turns them into often dangerous substitutes for genuine experience, and thus into mechanisms of escape from the reality and urgency of our indigenous problems.

[2] Jung, *Psychologie und Alchemie*, p. 19.

in and behind their lives which transcends their individual egos.

All this is not a question of deliberate choice but of a spontaneous psychic occurrence. This is proved most convincingly by the fact that there are not only those who want to find their way back to an established creed and nevertheless, in honesty to their inner experience, find it impossible to accept such a solution for themselves, but also those who feel the strongest possible resistance against accepting any "religious" solution of their problems and nevertheless find it forced on them by the strength of their inner experience. They are the "rational" people who come merely for the "removal" of some "silly" neurotic symptom, and to their horror have to discover that the cure lies in the acceptance of some "irrational" process in their psyche of which they had been unaware.[1]

All these people have one crucial point in common: they feel that only their immediate individual experience can be valid and obligatory for them. Thus they have to look inside instead of outside for a solution of their psychological problem, however it may manifest itself, whether it is immediately apparent as one of spiritual isolation and lack of inner relatedness, or whether it is only found later on to be so. To the three great virtues of faith, hope and love a fourth is thus added, out of the necessities of the situation and as an indispensable condition for any satisfactory answer—that of individual realization. This realization can only be achieved by an individual enquiry into the foundations of life, without reliance on historical and traditional statements. Such an enquiry represents a daring adventure, for it takes man out of all guaranteed security; yet it is not a "reckless adventure, but an effort inspired by deep spiritual distress to bring meaning once more into life on the basis of fresh and unprejudiced experience."[2]

In undertaking this adventure, all those people who are forced by the urgency of their psychological situation to find an answer

[1] As evidence for this cf. the case described on p. 76ff.
[2] Jung, *Modern Man in Search of a Soul*, p. 276.

to the question of the meaning of their lives are the expression
and the carriers of the problem of modern man. They are forced,
not out of a deliberate decision but out of an inner conflict
which has been developing for centuries, to seek a reconciliation
of the two poles of the non-ego and the ego. This conflict first
became apparent in the Renaissance, and has been growing in
intensity ever since.[1] It starts with the discovery of the importance of the *individual* and of individual *experience*. This
has gone hand in hand with a constantly growing withdrawal of
projections from the outside world and a corresponding realization of the inner conditions of man. It is only too obvious how
this withdrawal of projections has turned into a rejection of
everything that is not made by the ego; this creates a dangerous
identification of the inner conditions of man with the sphere
of the conscious mind. But we are coming to realize more and
more that the inner conditions of man include the pre-conscious
and supra-individual roots, and we are now looking within ourselves for their revelation instead of outside.

Whatever the dangerous consequences of the insistence on
the importance of the ego and of individual experience may
be, we have to realize that the power of the ego and of the
conscious mind, with all its doubts and its inquisitiveness, with
all its loss of relatedness and all its genuine curiosity, has grown
as an expression of man's process of individuation. On the one
hand, the ritual as a re-enactment of the original encounter with
the eternal numinosum is at least potentially infinitely greater
and more powerful than individual consciousness can ever be.
But on the other hand it is in the *hic et nunc*, in the here and
now, that the energy of the supra-individual and eternal images
becomes apparent. Timelessness, eternity, is not interested in the
present; it is a circle in which past and future merge into one
another without a break. It is individual consciousness which
stops the eternal flow for an infinitesimal second and becomes
the one reality which is the actualization of the eternal images.
Our individual presence lies between the eternal past and the

[1]For a more detailed analysis of this situation cf. the last essay in this volume:
"C. G. Jung's Contribution to Modern Consciousness."

eternal future; and this eternity has, as it were, to be re-interpreted by each individual if it is to yield its creative energy. In this process of re-interpretation each individual has to find his own relation to the eternal laws according to his individual capacity.

This puts quite a new and unique responsibility on each individual who, forced by his own experience, finds himself the interpreter of the eternal images, the archetypes. Unless his interpretation does justice to the substance of the archetypal images, their creative energy is lost, and with it the creative energy of man. If, on the other hand, the interpretation is adequate, then our conscious mind, our ego, is again brought into communication with our roots in the non-ego; our present is linked to the past, and the chain of existence is kept unbroken. The individual no longer feels isolated, and his existence gains a new meaning as the particular actualization of an eternal and supra-individual process of life.

If "a psycho-neurosis must be understood as the suffering of a human being who has not discovered what life means for him,"[1] then the discovery of the eternal images of meaning and significance, as most intensely expressed in the experience of the "self" as the archetype of the Deity, indeed means a cure. "To the patient it is nothing less than a revelation when, from the hidden depths of the psyche, something arises to confront him—something strange that is not the 'I' and is therefore beyond the reach of personal caprice. He has gained access to the sources of psychic life, and this marks the beginning of the cure."[2] One of my patients once formulated this experience in these words: "To me the real discovery of psychology has been that there is a sense which we don't make." And one may add: that this is a sense which these people find inside themselves, that it grows out of the emergency and urge of their situation.

In their "neurosis" the psychological crisis of our age becomes apparent, and in the solution that they find, men give at the same time a more than individually valid answer. The crisis is

[1] Jung, *Modern Man in Search of a Soul*, p. 260.
[2] Ibid., p. 280.

that of the split between life and meaning, and of the spiritual isolation which this causes. The answer—and in it a new synthesis—is that of the rediscovery by the individual of the numinous and supra-individual images as eternally present in our psyche and as its eternal foundation.[1] This answer is "based on a perception of the symbols of the unconscious individuation process, which always sets in when the ruling collective conceptions which govern human life fall into decay."[2] The individual's convincing experience of these supra-individual symbols means a new relatedness with and a new obligation towards the "religious" process in ourselves. It represents the synthesis between the ego and the non-ego, between the activities of the conscious and the unconscious psyche. This synthesis creates a new awareness which mediates between the two poles and forms the bridge between timeless eternity and the individual existence which is limited by time. While the unconscious is passive and the conscious psyche active, such awareness is "active passivity," i.e. a watchful turning in to the non-arbitrary emergence of the eternal images. Whereas the unconscious is on the side of unreflecting tradition and faith, and the conscious mind on the side of doubting rejection of tradition, and of faithlessness, this awareness is a reflecting acceptance and knowing faith arising out of the strength of the immediate inner experience. It can be defined as a growing "penetrability" for the eternal ideas and symbols; it is a progressive purification of the tools of inner perception (starting with the freeing of the ego from its pathological complexes and identifications) so that man becomes able to perceive the inner fate and meaning, until—in the process of integration—he may in the end become the immaculate channel between the infinite and the finite.

To use a metaphor, or rather a symbol, the conscious and the

---

[1] It is interesting to note that the discovery of primitive art (and also of the art of children) coincides with the formulation of modern psychology. As so often happens, the inner process first becomes apparent in a projection: "primitive" art exerts its fascination as the projection of "primitive" creativeness in ourselves, i.e. as an expression of the pre-conscious and primordial images in our psyche.

[2] Jung, *Psychologie und Alchemie*, p. 60.

unconscious psyche may be understood as the two poles or foci
of an ellipse, which both together define the shape of the curve.
When the distance between the two poles becomes infinite, that
is when the two poles are completely torn from one another, an
irremediable split has occurred and the content of the ellipse
is nil. But when the two poles become one, that is when complete harmonization has taken place, the result is the circle,
which is the ellipse with the greatest possible content. This corresponds to Jung's concept of the "self" which he defines as the
new centre of gravity that is the synthesis between the conscious
and the unconscious psyche. This self is the highest realization of
the individual, and at the same time transcends the individual
completely. It is the synthesis between the external and the internal reality. It is in me and I am in it. It is our goal, and at the
same time it is the source from which we came and which constantly feeds us. It is not possible to speak of it except in paradoxical terms because it is so much more than a logical conclusion or theoretical abstraction; it is living reality and experience.
It is "the god in us."[1] In religious language it would be called
the knowledge of the supreme importance of the human individual as the particular and decisive instance of the divine; or
it might be said that it is the divine that has become manifest
in man, and man who has become the actualization of the divine.
It is the knowledge of man's significance and responsibility for
the fulfilment of the fate of creation, as it is formulated in this
answer of a Hasidic rabbi to his pupils:

"Rabbi Elias was asked by one of his disciples: 'Rabbi, what
is the Messiah waiting for?' The Rabbi answered: 'For you.' "

APPENDIX TO PAGE 189

There is an interesting representation of this process in the symbolism of the Kabbalah. The Kabbalah talks of the ten sefiroth, or emanations of divine aspects. All these emanations emerge from what the
Kabbalists call the En-Sof, the Infinite who is hidden and impercep-

[1] Jung, *Two Essays on Analytical Psychology*, p. 265.

tible to anything but Himself. In the process of emanation the Infinite turns himself into Creation and Self-Revelation. En-Sof, the Infinite, is the inexpressible Fullness. In the process of Creation and Self-Revelation the Infinite externalizes Himself, and His light that has so far been shining only inwardly in Himself, is made visible. This stage is called by the Kabbalists the Nothingness. It is this mystical Nothingness, otherwise called the Kether Elyon, the supreme crown of the Deity, from which all the other stages of God's gradual unfolding in the sefiroth emanate. What the Kabbalists mean by this becomes clear through another metaphor they use: the Nothingness is the abyss which has become visible in the gaps of existence. Translated into psychological terms this means: En-Sof is the life-power beyond realization. Creation, Self-Revelation is analogous to the lightning of man's consciousness which at the same time reveals the unique split in his existence, that is the separation out of complete self-unawareness—"the abyss which has become visible in the gaps of existence." The next two sefiroth are those of Hokhmah and Binah, Wisdom and Intelligence. God's wisdom represents the ideal thought of Creation, and it is also called Reshith, the Beginning. In this wisdom the ideal existence of all things is, as it were, enshrined; it is still undeveloped and undifferentiated and therefore also called the "Point," but nevertheless the essence of all that exists is derived from this sefirah Hokhmah, wisdom. But in the next sefirah Binah, Intelligence, what has been hidden and was as it were folded up in the point is now unfolded. The name of this sefirah, Binah, has etymologically the same root as the word ben, between, and so Binah means the Intelligence which penetrates between things and divides them, that is differentiation, and discrimination. Whereas in the divine wisdom everything was still undifferentiated, its forms are now already preformed in Binah, the divine Intelligence. To later Kabbalists the two sefiroth of Hokhmah and Binah have become the potencies of Father and Mother, thus representing the two creative polarities from out of which everything else comes forth.[1]

[1]Cf. G. Scholem, *Major Trends in Jewish Mysticism*, Schocken, Jerusalem, 1941, p. 213ff.

VII

C. G. JUNG'S CONTRIBUTION TO MODERN CONSCIOUSNESS

NO DAY seems more fitting for assessing the achievement of a life than the seventieth birthday, with its symbolical significance of the completed span of human life. And C. G. Jung, with his appreciation of the symbol, will, I hope, forgive it if one of his pupils—who gladly and gratefully admits that contact with him has enriched his own life beyond recognition—tries to answer this question as far as his teacher's outward influence is concerned.

The question which seems the most important is this: what has C. G. Jung's life work meant to modern man; what is his contribution to modern consciousness, and what obligation results from his teaching? For Jung—like Freud—has by his genius far transcended the limited domain of psychiatry, and has immensely widened the scope of psychology; he has thus become an interpreter of our human situation as a whole. Psychology has proved to be the new instrument for understanding and defining the human situation where religion and philosophy have lost their hold and power. Thus psychology is not just another specialized branch of science—its very existence, and the intensity of its impact, are the expression and the measure of a new phase in human development.

Nobody has been more aware of the spiritual obligation implied in psychology than C. G. Jung. To him the fact of his Swiss birth has always been more than a mere coincidence; it is the symbolical expression of his central position in Europe. He has held and administered the passes between north and south; he has lived in the very centre of Europe where three different cultures and languages meet; and from this central position he has reached beyond the Channel and the Atlantic. It is interesting to know that even the English language and English culture came to him in Switzerland; for two years, during 1917 and 1918, he was in charge of the British prisoners of war interned in Château d'Oex. Ever since, his contact with the Anglo-American world has been close, so much so that even most of his seminars have been in English. It has always been his aim to find a true synthesis of all these different trends of European civilization—their centre, and indeed the "self" of Europe.

The task which his awareness of the spiritual obligation of psychology has imposed on Jung has been no easy one. It has led to much ill-founded criticism and misunderstanding of his intentions. One of the chief things to which objection has been taken is Jung's so-called mystical trend. But his sense of spiritual obligation has meant to Jung the necessity of synthesizing the divergent lines of European—and not only European—spiritual history. Nobody has realized more keenly the deep cleavage in the European soul and has given a more cogent analysis of it than Jung. To him modern man is not the isolated and self-sufficient product of modern times, but the sum total of the history of a European process of individuation. That explains why, starting from modern psychiatry, he has gradually worked his way back into the origins of modern European psychology, and has indeed gone far beyond Europe itself, in an attempt to discover the undertones and hidden trends and urges of this process.

In this essay an attempt will be made to sketch the historical line and background of our modern European psychological situation, and thus to show Jung's place and function in the development of the modern mind. In itself this interpretation is naturally based on the concepts of Analytical Psychology. Thus the following attempt to trace the development of modern consciousness, to show the conflict inherent in it, and to point out

Jung's contribution to a solution of it, is in itself a presentation of Jung's thought; without it, it could never have been undertaken.

The question that immediately arises is this: What is meant by the phrase "modern European mind"? What is the specific position of modern consciousness, what is this modern "*Weltbild,*" the image of the world that seems so brimful of conflicts and potentialities, of conflicts which have led Europe into its deepest crisis, and at the same time may be fore-runners of a new and more adult phase of its life?

The origins of what we call "modern consciousness" and "modern man"[1] can be traced back to the Renaissance. It was the Renaissance which created a conception of man and his world which was fundamentally different from that of the Middle Ages. It is this change-over from an old image of man and world to the new "modern" one which has created both the immense possibilities of development and the equally immense dangers of destruction which have come out so clearly in our days.

The medieval conception of the world and of man's rôle in it was fundamentally different from that of modern man. It was uniform, collective, and static as against the individual and dynamic conception that is modern man's. The individual as such did not play any significant rôle. As Jacob Burckhardt has pointed out, "man was conscious of himself only through some general category," be it "as member of a race, people, party, family, or corporation."[2] Each of these social categories was accepted as the expression of a natural, that is, a divine, order. The individual who could choose his own conditions

---

[1]The term "modern man" will be used in a double sense. First, it is used in a historical sense in the same way as in the expression "modern history." In this sense the history of modern man starts with the end of the Middle Ages. Secondly, it is used to describe the result of this historical development. It is in this second sense that Jung uses the term e.g. in his essay, "The Spiritual Problem of Modern Man" (in *Modern Man in Search of a Soul*). There he defines "modern man" as "the man of the immediate present" (loc. cit., p. 227).

[2]Jacob Burckhardt, *The Civilization of the Renaissance in Italy*, Phaidon Edition, London, 1944, p. 81.

and aims did not yet exist. "In having a distinct, unchangeable, and unquestionable place in the social world from the moment of birth, man was rooted in a structuralized whole, and thus life had a meaning which left no place, and no need, for doubt."[1] These collective ties, with their inherent lack of freedom, were undoubtedly often felt to be irksome, but man received in return an immense compensation for these limitations: the clear definition of his position and function.

The needs of man were provided for in every respect. He was woven into a close texture of existence by which he and his life were clearly defined and contained. He lived securely protected in the bosom of the Church "outside which there is no salvation." No better or clearer symbol for man in this state could be found than that of his reliance and dependence upon *"ecclesia mater."* This great mother surrounded and nourished him. All the characteristics of the mother archetype can be found in the thought of that time.

Another characteristic of this psychological attitude was the static order of the world. This order went back to divine revelation and therefore was absolutely indisputable. No change in the conception of the universe was possible or indeed desirable. For this static and indisputable order of the universe made life and the world easy to understand. For medieval man "the earth was eternally fixed and at rest in the centre of the universe, encircled by the course of a sun that solicitously bestowed its warmth. Men were all children of God under the loving care of the Most High, who prepared them for eternal blessedness; and all knew exactly what they should do and how they should conduct themselves in order to rise from a corruptible world to an incorruptible and joyous existence."[2]

The psychological problem involved in this state of mind is obvious. It is just that of the manifest non-existence of the

---

[1] Erich Fromm, *The Fear of Freedom*, Kegan Paul, London, 1942, p. 34. Although the approach of this book is different from the one attempted here, the analysis leads nevertheless to a very similar description of the psychological situation.

[2] Jung, *Modern Man in Search of a Soul*, p. 235.

individual. This non-existence does not necessarily mean that the concept of individuality was merely "repressed"; it is more likely that it had not yet reached the threshold of consciousness of the average man of the time. In other words, the concept of individuality was still subliminal. This manifest absence of individuality conforms to the domination by the mother archetype. It expresses itself in a state of more or less complete *"participation mystique,"* in identity with the collective organism, and the rejection of the discriminating "masculine" functions of the psyche. It is conservative and traditional, and close to the instincts.

In this psychological state, which is characterized by its "feminine" and passive features, the "masculine" and active ones are unconscious. But one of the fundamental laws of psychic energy is that of enantiodromia. Jung has made use of this term, "to describe the emergence of the unconscious opposite, with particular relation to its chronological sequence. This characteristic phenomenon occurs almost universally wherever an extreme, one-sided tendency dominates the conscious life; for this involves the gradual development of an equally strong, unconscious counter-position, which first becomes manifest in an inhibition of conscious activities, and subsequently leads to an interruption of conscious direction."[1]

For a very long time these opposite psychic tendencies had no chance of emerging. Whatever traces of a growing individuality there may have been, as far as their manifestations went, the authority of *"ecclesia mater"* and her dogma was able to keep it underground. But in this restrictive attitude the Church was forced to become more and more rigid. It was just this rigidity which in the end made her authority too brittle to work successfully. The attempt to suppress forces which the Church felt to be a danger to her dogmatic, "catholic," and "all-embracing" conception of the world and man's rôle in it was besides never wholly successful. Even if these forces had not yet become manifestly effective, they nevertheless led an

[1] Jung, *Psychological Types*, p. 542.

increasingly strong and fertile underground existence.[1] They had, as it were, played the rôle of an "autonomous complex" in the psyche of the "mother."

It would, of course, go beyond the framework of the present essay to go into the history of these "underground movements" of individuality. But their general trend, which may be comprised under the name of "gnosis"[2] and which is closely connected with the history of heresy (heresy means, characteristically enough, "an act of choosing"), is clearly enough that of emphasizing the individual and discriminating experience as against the dogmatic and collectively obligatory statement.

With the Renaissance these subliminal forces became visibly and manifestly potent. The "theocentric" conception of the world was rapidly breaking up in favour of an "anthropocentric" one. Besides laying emphasis on the importance of the individual experience, the main characteristics of this conception were its dynamic, discriminating and intellectual character. All these characteristics are typical of a predominantly "masculine" attitude. Whereas the feminine attitude is characterized, among other things, by its emphasis on the personal values, through the predominance of the feeling function,[3] the masculine attitude is characterized by its emphasis on objective facts as expressed in the thinking function. Thus the medieval attitude had been directed towards establishing man's subjective position, whereas the attitude of the Renaissance was directed towards the establishment of objective laws.[4] Perhaps the most striking expression

[1] It must not be overlooked that in spite of the manifestly collective character of the Middle Ages the germ of the individual attitude is inherent just in the Christian conception of immortality. The idea that each individual possesses an immortal soul is the foundation of individuation. It is this very germ which has finally blossomed out into the self-discovery of the individual.

[2] An important disguise of the gnostic heresy was Alchemy (cf. Jung, *Psychology and Religion*, p. 108).

[3] Cf. Jung, *Psychological Types*, p. 543: "Feeling is primarily a process that takes place between the ego and a given content, a process, moreover, that imparts to the content a definite *value* in the sense of acceptance or rejection ('like' or 'dislike')."

[4] Of course, this does not mean that the intellectual approach had been non-existent during the Middle Ages. But its function and direction had been fundamentally different from that of a later time. Thus the supreme intellect of a

and symbol of the change in the spiritual image of the world is found in the discoveries of Copernicus. The destruction of the geocentric conception of the world and the establishment of the heliocentric one—which is the counterpart on the plane of natural science to the anthropocentric conception—throws man back on himself. The world and its order are no longer indisputable but open to discussion and subject to changes. Man's earth is no longer the hub and the destination of the universe.[1] Instead of being a strictly defined part of a general world-order man discovers, and has to rely upon, his individual consciousness as the determining factor in his life. This fact together with the growing emphasis on the importance of experience leads to the development of all the "discriminating" energies and so to the emancipation of the intellect. This means the most positive and creative discovery of modern man: the scientific and experimental attitude and the insistence on experience.

At the same time, however, the development of individuality and of science was bound to create a psychological problem of tremendous proportions. Had there been only a creative and progressive side to modern consciousness, our modern crisis would not be understandable. The real psychological problem lies in the ambivalence of the new step in human consciousness. The development of the individual attitude leads to the loss of collective security; the development of all the discriminating energies leads, and led only too easily, to an attitude of general scepticism; that of the enquiring attitude to one of general

---

Thomas Aquinas was directed towards establishing the laws of a universal *"ordo"* of the world, of a hierarchical order of existence whose last justification rested in God, and in which each individual found his befitting place. To St. Thomas the "two orders of nature and supernature—the first the object of reason, the other of Faith—are in reality one, owing their unity and cohesion to the one God from whom all proceeds and to whom all tends. . . . Hence all St. Thomas's thought centres in God, and all science, however 'secular,' receives a religious significance." His system is "based on eternal and unchangeable theological and metaphysical principles, and as such quite independent of the data of physical sciences and experiment." (Rev. V. White, O.P.: *Scholasticism*, Catholic Truth Society, London, pp. 24 and 26).

[1] Giordano Bruno's philosophy, especially his idea of the innumerable inhabited worlds, represents the final end of the geocentric conception.

doubt. Whereas before the maternal, feminine, feeling forces had established the subjective values of man, this situation was now fundamentally changed through the new conceptions.

For instance, as Burckhardt[1] has pointed out, the mental attitude of the Renaissance promoted "the dissolution of the most essential dogmas of Christianity." Foremost among these were the ideas of immortality and salvation. As a matter of fact, for the Middle Ages—the "theological period" of mankind as Comte calls it—the main interest lay in the salvation of the soul, and man's rôle in the universe was expressed by this task. With the transition from the geocentric to the heliocentric conception of the universe, man's interest seems to have shifted away completely from his own person to nature. And suddenly, with this shifting of the interest from the earth to the universe, the idea of salvation lost its significance.

Obviously the old conceptions, as long as they were accepted, that means felt, by man, were bound to give him a great sense of confidence and security. Now this very security was taken away by the new ideas. Man had been freed from a stifling limitation, but had received in exchange an enormous burden of which he only gradually became aware. With the decline in the belief in immortality man had more and more lost interest in the problem of his own soul. The main interest lay outside, and "inside" was no longer a problem worthy of the attention of a scientific mind. Life had become a merely biological-physiological phenomenon that obeyed mechanical laws, whereas the question of value and meaning was the domain of the despised or condescendingly tolerated "unscientific" mind.

It was the conflict between "faith" and "knowledge"—a conflict which had been so much the theme of the heretics and the "gnosis"—that had come into the open. A characteristic figure in this conflict is Paracelsus, and it is for this reason that Jung has been deeply interested in his person and teaching.[2] Paracelsus is one of the most important figures of the movement

1 Loc. cit., p. 339.
2Cf. Jung, *Paracelsica*.

of the Renaissance in Northern Europe. In him both the forces of the Middle Ages and the Renaissance were alive and creative. To establish the autonomy and independence of scientific experience as against the authority of tradition without destroying the specific values of the latter is the fundamental theme of Paracelsus's thought.[1] He accepted the binding character of the divine revelation with regard to religion and faith, but he could not accept it as obligatory for the study of nature. Here he relied on the *"lumen naturae"* which was to him a second and independent source of cognition in addition to the divine revelation. Paracelsus's disciple, Adam von Bodenstein, wrote: "The student of nature has the matters of nature not through authority, but through his own experience."[2]

This distinction between knowledge given through revelation and knowledge given through individual experience, with both its polarity and its inherent conflict, finds a parallel in the psychological distinction between the non-ego and the ego. The ego is the centre, and the representative, of the conscious mind. The sum of psychic energy which is disposable to the conscious mind is what we call "will."[3] This concept of the ego hardly needs any further explanation. Much more complicated, however, and leading straight into the specific field of Analytical Psychology, is Jung's concept of the non-ego. The total personality consists of conscious *and* unconscious components. Among the unconscious components the "repressed" contents represent only a limited and relatively unimportant part. They are derived from the conscious part of the psyche and are thus not essentially different from it. Those contents of the unconscious which are essentially distinct from the conscious—and these are the most important—are not due to repressions. This means that they do not have their origin in the conscious mind, but, on the contrary, have existed before consciousness: "The conscious mind is based upon, and results from, an unconscious psyche which is prior to con-

[1] Ibid., pp. 50ff.
[2] Ibid., p. 47.
[3] Cf. Jung, *Psychological Types*, p. 616.

sciousness and continues to function together with, or despite, consciousness."[1] Jung has defined this "unconscious psyche which is prior to consciousness" as the "collective unconscious," and its manifestations as the "archetypes." It is this collective unconscious which is not ego, and as it is not derived from the ego either, it is also non-ego. It has not only existed before consciousness, but is "the mother of consciousness."[2]

Although the conscious mind and its representative and centre, the ego, form the typical human achievement, this achievement is also a danger through its exclusiveness and distance from the instinctive foundations. Whereas, therefore, the conscious mind and the ego (and will) are absolutely necessary for the creation of the subject which is to perceive the images of the collective unconscious, the non-ego is equally necessary to the working of the ego as a constant objective balance and regulation. In this sense the "subjective psyche"—the ego—and the "objective psyche"— the collective unconscious—stand in a compensatory relationship. The aim of the process of individuation is the creation of the centre common to both, and this centre Jung has called the self.

The ego has all the characteristics of transitoriness whereas the non-ego has the quality of "eternity," or of relative timelessness.[3] "The limits of the conscious mind can be defined; the unconscious, however, is the unknown psyche *per se* and as such unlimited because undefinable."[4] For that reason it has numinous character, and is the carrier of tremendous psychic energy. That is why the experience of the non-ego is perceived as "God." And such "he personifies the collective unconscious which has not yet been integrated into human realization."[5] The ego possesses more or less complete control over its manifestations through the will; it is the unknown and unlimited energy of the objective psyche which is beyond the control of the

---

[1]Jung, *The Integration of the Personality*, p. 13.
[2]Ibid., p. 12.
[3]Jung, *Psychologie und Alchemie*, p. 155.
[4]Ibid., pp. 253f.
[5]Jung, *Das Göttliche Kind*, p. 104.

subject. The subject can either relate to or reject the manifestations of the objective psyche. In the first case a growing integration of these manifestations into consciousness takes place and the *"homo totus,"*[1] the whole and undividuated personality whose centre is the self, is the result. In the second case, that of rejection, however, a split between the two parts of the psyche occurs, with negative results to the normal and constructive working of the psyche.

In Paracelsus's thought the two sources of cognition: divine revelation and the *"lumen naturae,"* did not represent a conflict, as both originated in the "unity of God."[2] To him the "self," as the centre of and constant mediator between the two, was still a living reality. But it is exactly this conflict between the two which became more and more marked, until, under the impact of the movement of "Enlightenment," in the nineteenth century the two poles, both originally essential parts of one united whole, finally assumed the position of deadly enemies. Paracelsus was still able to say: "I under the Lord, the Lord under me: I under him; outside my charge, and he under me: outside his charge"[3]—but the "I under the Lord" was to lose more and more of its obligation and meaning.

This process, it is true, remained for a considerable time more or less unconscious. It was still possible for such a great scientist as Newton to be equally interested in theology and mysticism. To a later age it appeared almost incredible, or could only be understood as the fancy of a genius, that the same man who "had conceived a working universe wholly independent of the spiritual order"[4] should also have written books on theology or, still worse, have been deeply engrossed in alchemical research.[5] But it shows how at that time religion and

---

[1] Jung, *Psychologie und Alchemie*, p. 17.
[2] Cf. Jung, *Paracelsica*, p. 52.
[3] Ibid., p. 52.
[4] Charles Singer, *A Short History of Science*, Clarendon Press, Oxford, 1941, p. 254.
[5] Cf. John Read, *Prelude to Chemistry*, Bell, London, 1939, p. 307f.: ". . . he had set himself to discover the Elixir of Life, and how to transmute base metals into gold. He was more than usually secretive about these romantic pursuits. . . . The Alchemy that Newton practised had more than its vocabulary in common with

science could still live side by side without an open clash.

The split between "knowledge" and "faith" had, however, widened more and more under the surface, and it was finally revealed in its full significance through the French Enlightenment, which owed so much to English empiricism. Voltaire— and the Encyclopaedists—expounded Newton's theory of physics to inaugurate a new phase of scepticism and materialism. Whereas in Newton the two sides—science and religion—had still existed side by side, the philosophy of Enlightenment killed the one by means of the other.

The psychological result of this growing split between knowledge and faith was most disturbing. The rejection of the religious interpretation and valuation of life and the world by more and more people meant also that to them the world no longer appeared as a spiritual and meaningful entity. That explains why, side by side with the great new discoveries and the progress of individual experience, there grew up a general feeling of insecurity and isolation. The "experimental" attitude meant that man was able, and indeed obliged, to question everything; and this attitude was bound to lead step by step to a growing feeling of doubt and scepticism. No longer was a comprehensive and acceptable answer given to the question of the meaning and significance of man's life. The more the laws that govern nature became visible, the more the laws that govern man's rôle in this world seemed to become blurred. The synthesizing spiritual principle that had been the characteristic of an earlier epoch had been lost, and man experienced the world merely in a bewildering variety of material aspects. The unity of life and meaning had been finally split. Man had lost his dignity as the exponent and function of a meaningful world. The last and most pathetic expression of this attitude is the one which regards man as significant only as an "economic unit."

The twentieth century thus shows a devastating sense of

mysticism, and no doubt it was by way of Alchemy that Newton entered upon the Interpretation of the Prophecies which forms so large a part of his Theological writings." (Quotation from the foreword to the "Catalogue of the Newton Papers," Sotheby & Co., London, 1936.)

frustration and futility in the image of the world as seen by the average man. It can be defined as something like this: the world is without divine direction; it is without immanent sense or inner coherence (except the purely mechanical one); it is without intrinsic responsibility. This means that man has no reality or function in this world beyond the one that his ego defines for himself.

The tremendous and in itself invaluable achievement of the rational and experimental attitude had begun by freeing man from an enormous number of inhibiting bonds and had disposed of the limitations of dogmatic authority. The motto of the Royal Society, *"Nullius in verba"* (on the word of no man), expresses the justified pride of this new discovery of man's freedom to doubt and enquire; but intellect had apparently overreached itself; it had not only attacked wrong dogmas but also legitimate values. Intellect had assumed the rôle of the panacea instead of limiting itself to its proper place and function. Human values are not open to rationalistic dissection; the laws of intellect are different from those of feeling.

The development of the intellectual and rational approach was a necessary and creative step in the development and differentiation of the human psyche. Every differentiation, however, carries with it a certain onesidedness. In a relatively undifferentiated state more things are perceived but in a relatively dimmer and more diffuse way. Differentiation means concentration on comparatively few contents which are perceived in a clearer and more sharply defined way. Such differentiation goes with a development of the will. Primitive man—and children—cannot rely on their will, which is a function of the established ego. Necessary as the ego is as an instrument of human achievement, it also produces new mistakes and conflicts through its exclusiveness and onesidedness. "With the growing differentiation of the will there exists a correspondingly greater danger of an aberration into onesidedness and of a digression into a lawless and rootless state. On the one hand this represents the possibility of human freedom, on the other hand, however, it is also the source of endless sins against the instinct. . . . The more the conscious mind becomes differentiated the greater also becomes the danger of being separated from its roots."[1] This state of being cut off from the instinctive roots necessarily produces a deep feeling of isolation and insecurity and thus of frustration.

As was to be expected, this feeling of insecurity and frustration has produced two opposite escape mechanisms. The one is a regression into a previous state of consciousness, the other a repression of the problem. The first resulted in a rejection of the scientific and intellectual attitude and led to a fatal surrender to collective and irrational values. This surrender had been foreshadowed in the romantic movement with its sentimental insistence on the infinite and transcendental. The heritage of this movement was an inevitable regression inasmuch as it meant a complete renunciation of the new achievement of the human mind, namely of the differentiated ego and the rational approach. Every such loss of the one pole of the psyche, however, leads to an unconscious identification with the other. A complete loss of balance and dissociation is the result, and this produces a quasi-psychotic state. The lost energy of the repressed side reappears in the unconscious, and like every unconscious content becomes projected into a suitable object. The tragic results of this romantic regression have become only too obvious to all of us: Fascism and the *"Blut und Boden"* myth, where the lost energy of the ego reappeared in the projection on to the Duce and Führer, are its direct descendants. They are tragic infantile misunderstandings of the human need for the non-rational.

Equally futile and disastrous has been the attempt to deny and cover up the problems that had come into being as the heritage of the Renaissance. The short-lived pseudo-philosophical bubble of "evolutionary progress" only served to show up even more clearly the futility of man's thought about himself and the meaning of his life. The romantic regression meant a surrender to the non-rational side which had to be paid for by the sacrifice of the rational and individual side. The repression of the con-

[1] Jung, *Das Göttliche Kind*, pp. 100ff.

flict between intellect and feeling, between masculine and feminine values, on the other hand produced a devitalized and mechanized world. All non-rational and feeling-values—religion, love, art—lost their numinous character; instead of presenting man with the fullness and depth of life, instead of being a constant obligation and challenge, they had become niceties and pretexts. Religion no longer knew of the *"deus absconditus,"* but was turned into a system of collective ethical behaviour; love became an empty shell of sentimental hypocrisy and lies; art was no longer looked upon as a living influence in human life. The nineteenth century became the era of "respectability" and anaemic ideals. Instead of the challenge of religion, collective rules of behaviour; instead of the fullness of love, sentimentality; instead of the obligation of art, the enjoyment of aesthetic shadows—this was the tragi-comic result of the gigantic undertaking of the Renaissance. Only in science itself did the heritage of the Renaissance produce its full blossom.

But just as the repressions that went with the increasing dogmatism and formalism of the Middle Ages had produced the enantiodromiacal reaction of the Renaissance, so the repressions of the age of materialism and respectability produced its deadly challenge out of itself. Kierkegaard, Nietzsche, and Freud are the three devastating critics of the nineteenth century, which is their origin and which determined their fate.

In Kierkegaard the nineteenth century found the expression of its profoundest reaction against the formalism and utilitarianism of its religious decadence. He was fully aware of the tragic feeling of isolation and futility that was the deepest wound of his age. While everybody else tried to look away from it he had the heroic courage to probe deeply into this feeling of being lost in a hostile world. In him the unbridgeable gap between this world and God, between faith and knowledge, found its most intense expression. "We are always in the wrong in relation to God." Here is the tragic paradox between life that is meant to possess a profound meaning and direction, and its actuality which always falls short of that meaning. Knowledge is bound to fail man; his attempt to understand is futile and without hope of accomplishment. Intellectual thought always comes up against insoluble paradoxes; only impassioned faith can transcend this essential tragedy of human life.

Where Kierkegaard's reaction to the problem of the nineteenth century had been that of insistence on the complete powerlessness of man, Nietzsche, not less critical of his time than the great Dane, went to the other extreme. To him the empty moral values of the nineteenth century are the "judgments of tired men"; it is the strongest affects and emotions which are the sources of power. Into the nineteenth century with its shallow ideals and its belief in utilitarian progress he throws his challenge of the superman. "He who no longer finds the great in God, does not find it at all—he has to deny it or to create it."

Nietzsche's "Superman" and his concept of the death of God ("*Gott ist tot*") represented the climax in a development which goes back to the origins of modern consciousness. Before the men of the Renaissance had started their adventure in science, and in it discovered the objective laws of nature, this very nature had been the dwelling-place of every possible projection. The process of withdrawing these projections had already started with Christianity which had killed the Olympic gods and the anthropomorphic projections which they carried. But nature had still been full of spirits and demons of every description. It was left to modern science to de-spiritualize nature completely; the demons disappeared from nature to the same degree as its objective laws were explored. Science and experiment thus put an end to the mythical identity of man and surrounding nature. Nature had become a mechanical and predictable quantity.[1]

But something else that was to prove of far-reaching consequence had happened with and through this de-spiritualization of nature. Projections, however unconscious and deceptive they may be, nevertheless fulfil an important need of the human psyche. What I don't know about myself, I find in somebody or something else. If this somebody or something else can for

[1] Cf. Jung, *Psychology and Religion*, pp. 100ff.

some reason or other no longer hold my projections, the projected content is thrown back on myself.

This is exactly what has happened to modern man to an ever increasing degree. The gods and demons that could no longer hold their abode in the field of the physicists were discovered to have retreated into the human psyche. Instead of nature being full of gods and demons it was the human psyche that had to contain them all. A terrifying vitalization of the human psyche was the result. Instead of Olympus and Hades which had been lost to man, the unconscious mind was discovered. For the powers that man had unwillingly been forced to sacrifice outside himself he found no mean counter-balance in his own psyche.[1]

Nietzsche's intuitive genius formulated this idea in his words: "God is dead." He denied God—and at the same time re-created him in his Superman. Man to him had to become the new god; thus he identified the ego completely with god. This deification of the ego and the hypertrophy of the conscious mind led to such an inflation that the unconscious became more and more antagonistic; and it finally burst the dams.[2] Nietzsche became the self-sacrificing victim of his realization—Dionysus Zagreus, as he signed himself during his illness, who "was cut to pieces by the murderous knives of his enemies."[3]

In his attempt to deify man, Nietzsche had "decided to reject the snake and the 'ugliest man' and thus to expose himself to a heroic constraint of consciousness that led consistently to the collapse"[4] which he himself had foretold in his *Zarathustra*. Significantly enough it was not the philosopher but the doctor who at last dared descend into the dark depths of the instinctive drives and was thus finally to destroy the utilitarian illusions and sentimental hypocrisies of the nineteenth century.

Freud is the "great destroyer who bursts the shackles of the

---

[1]Cf. Jung, *Das Wandlungssymbol in der Messe*, Eranos Jahr-Buch, 1940–41, pp. 120f.
[2]Jung, *The Integration of the Personality*, p. 125.
[3]Frazer, *The Golden Bough*, Macmillan, London, 1926, Vol. VII, p. 13.
[4]Jung, *The Integration of the Personality*, p. 160.

past.''[1] His is the passionate power of the period of Enlightenment. Everything has to be "unmasked." He reveals the repressions and over-compensations of a basically cowardly civilization which was in deadly fear of its own instincts. He is the indigenous critic and conqueror of an era of repressions and illusions. He is—together with Nietzsche—the rediscoverer of the human instincts.

But he is also conditioned and limited by his own era. Its shallowness and self-deceits can be traced back to the exaggerations and illicit intrusions of the intellectual and rationalistic attitudes. The former he destroyed conclusively, the latter still held him under their spell. His attitude is still mainly that of the scientific materialism of the nineteenth century. His psychological approach is essentially biological. In his quest to unmask the illusions of the nineteenth century and to reveal the repressions behind their religious, moral and artistic—in short their spiritual—values he does not seem to see that these values have been misused. What he fights are distortions which served as mechanisms of escape, and in this process he overlooks the fact that behind these distortions there are genuine and creative impulses of the human psyche. It is as if he kills the disease but with it also the living organism on which it develops.

Like Nietzsche he is an answer to the disease of the nineteenth century,[2] and without the realization of this disease, without the realization of the falsehood of its values, there could be no way out of the sterile impasse. That is why Freud's approach had to be essentially reductive and analytical, as pseudo-ideals and fake-values had to be reduced to their true biological drives. But in this general process of unmasking, the distinction between genuine spiritual values and their falsification had also been destroyed.[3] The true values had become involved in this process, and man appeared completely defined by the fate of his biological drives.

[1] Jung, *Wirklichkeit der Seele*, p. 123.
[2] Ibid., p. 125.
[3] In this connection the similar rôle of Marx and "historical materialism" has to be mentioned.

The very fact, however, that psychology had become the concern of modern man shows that in it he instinctively felt the possibility of an answer to his so long repressed quest for the meaning of his life. His interest in psychology is "symptomatic of a profound convulsion of spiritual life."[1] Material interests had almost completely saturated man's needs for a long period —as long in fact as the original drive of the freed energy could still flow unimpeded by doubt. As long as the claim of science to be the guarantor of continuous progress still seemed to have some justification, the inner doubts and needs could be silenced. But when the limitations of progress in the external world became only too obvious—and whoever had not noticed anything before was rudely awakened by the first world war—man began to turn away from it and back to himself. "The rapid and world-wide growth of a 'psychological' interest over the last two decades[2] shows unmistakably that modern man has to some extent turned his attention from material things to his own subjective processes. . . . This 'psychological' interest of the present time shows that man expects something from psychic life which he has not received from the outer world."[3]

Freud neither could nor would give an answer to the question of the meaning of man's life. To him human life was a continuous conflict between the dark untamed passions of the "Id" and the restricting influence of the "Ego." As he said himself (in *Beyond the Pleasure Principle*) "the development of man needed no explanation that differed from that of the animals." No sentence could show more clearly than this how much Freud was still conditioned by the materialistic and rationalistic attitude of the nineteenth century. It is exactly at this point that Jung comes into his own.

After a short way in common with Freud, Jung soon began to see that the results of his research no longer allowed him to accept Freud's concept of the libido as valid. To Freud libido

[1] Jung, *Modern Man in Search of a Soul*, p. 233.
[2] This was written in 1928.
[3] Ibid., p. 237.

had been practically equivalent to the sexual urges, and the development of the personality was closely determined by the growing degree to which the ego could cope with them. Jung soon became convinced that the libido was not sufficiently defined by the sexual urges but that the concept of the libido had to be enlarged. To him libido became psychic energy in general, of which sexual urges represented only one, albeit an important, part. The experience which he acquired in his work with patients made it impossible for him to accept the materialistic, biological attitude of psychoanalysis for which spirit was a mere epiphenomenon produced by a doubtful process of sublimation. Thus he set out, in his *Psychology of the Unconscious,* to show how the libidinous process worked, as it were, in a dichotomous way—as instinctual (in the narrower sense) and as spiritual dynamism, whose common source was the psychic energy. Or as he expressed it almost thirty years after the first publication of the *Psychology of the Unconscious:* "Nature is not only matter, but it is also spirit."[1]

With that the unconscious received a completely different definition from that which it had been given by Freud. To Freud the unconscious was essentially defined by the "repressed" contents. Looked at from the point of view of the ego the unconscious according to Freud can on account of these repressed contents be regarded as the infantile *per se.* To Jung, however, the unconscious is "not merely a 'subconscious' appendix and still less a mere refuse-bin of the conscious mind, but on the contrary a largely autonomous psychic system which on the one hand functionally compensates the errors and onesidednesses of the conscious mind, and on the other hand, if necessary, corrects them forcibly."[2] In this sense, "the unconscious transcends the conscious mind and anticipates in its symbols future conscious processes. For this reason it is just as much a 'super-conscious.' "[3]

The symbols which are produced in the analytical process,

[1] Jung, *Paracelsica,* p. 170.
[2] Ibid., p. 171.
[3] Ibid.

"that is in the dialectical argument between the conscious and the unconscious,"[1] make the conclusion imperative that there exists in the psyche "an *a priori* potentiality of wholeness," a "wholeness which transcends the conscious mind."[2] Jung has given it also the name of the "self." It transcends the conscious mind in as far as it is the centre between the conscious and the unconscious, or between the ego and the non-ego (cf. above, p. 214f.).

The unconscious—as well as the self—is *a priori* existent, and the ego (and the conscious mind) are derived from it. "The self is an unconscious preformation of the ego. Not I create myself, but rather I happen to myself."[3] On the other hand, the ego is free and autonomous.[4] This is the essential antinomy of human existence. "In the reality of life both are always existent: the preponderance of the non-ego and the hypertrophy of the ego."[5] The ego stands to the self as the patiens to the agens,[6] and the process of individuation is really a process by which the ego becomes more and more aware of its relationship to the non-ego. With the growing realization of this relationship, the self can assume more and more of its function as the centre —and therefore as the *"unio oppositorum"*—of the total man.

This realization has finally led Jung to say that "the psyche is *'naturaliter religiosa,'* that is that it possesses a religious function."[7] In the face of a good deal of misunderstanding it should be clearly understood that Jung has not come to this formulation from "religious prejudices" or metaphysical speculations, but that it is merely the conclusion forced upon him by an unprejudiced evaluation of his material; in other words, that his approach is completely empirical. Jung has published a great wealth of clinical material which shows how a "religious" process is constantly at work in the human psyche. "Religious symbols

[1] Jung, *Psychologie und Alchemie*, p. 14.
[2] Jung, *Das Göttliche Kind*, p. 103.
[3] Jung, *Das Wandlungssymbol in der Messe*, p. 138.
[4] Ibid., p. 129.
[5] Ibid., p. 139.
[6] Ibid., p. 138.
[7] Jung, *Psychologie und Alchemie*, p. 26.

are manifestations of life, plain facts, and not intellectual opinions."[1] This religious process is simply the "process of individuation" i.e. "the psychological process that makes of a human being an 'individual'—a unique, indivisible unit or 'whole man.' "[2] It is religious in as far as it is concerned with the question of, and the quest for, the meaning of life. Where Freud sees the human life precariously balanced between the "Scylla of allowing and the Charybdis of forbidding," Jung finds in it "a development, a progression towards an aim or goal."[3] This process, whose nature also justifies the application of the concept of "entelechy," with its constantly progressing shift of the balance from the ego to the self as the centre of the personality, enables the latter to act as the "uniting symbol," in which the psychic conflicts are reconciled.

This uniting symbol as the carrier of the most powerful energy corresponds to the realization of "God" in religion. "That psychological fact which is the greatest power in your system is the god, since it is always the overwhelming psychic factor which is called god."[4] In order to grasp Jung's concept correctly, it is necessary to realize that when he talks about the "self," or the "uniting symbol," he is wholly concerned with *psychological* facts and factors. Psychology has neither the intention nor the power to discuss the absolute existence or non-existence of a god; it is only concerned with "god" as a psychological experience. "Psychology as the science of the psyche has to limit itself to its subject matter and has to guard itself against trespassing on metaphysical assertions or other statements of faith. Were it to postulate god even only as a hypothetical cause, it would imply the possibility of evidence for the existence of god, and by that it would have exceeded its competence in an absolutely illegitimate way. Science can only be science; there are no 'scientific' statements of faith and similar

[1] Jung, *The Integration of the Personality*, p. 144.
[2] Ibid., p. 3.
[3] Jung, *Psychologie und Alchemie*, p. 14.
[4] Jung, *Psychology and Religion*, p. 98.

contradictiones in adjecto. We just do not know what is the origin of the archetype, just as little as we know what is the origin of the psyche. The competence of psychology as an empirical science can only be to establish whether a typical image of the psyche can, by means of comparative research, justifiably be called an 'image of god' or not. This does not mean either a positive or negative statement with regard to the existence of god."[1]

Jung has seen himself forced on the strength of the evidence of his empirical psychological material to maintain the existence of such an "archetypal experience" which by all ages and civilizations has been formulated as "god." But the decisive difference between the approach of psychology and that of theology is this—that "for the former the religious figures refer to the self; whereas for the latter the self refers to its own central idea."[2] Just as it would be a serious mistake to mix up the experience of the archetype "god" with the absolute existence of god, however, it would be equally mistaken to assume that the fact of the psychological experience needs the depreciative qualification of the word "merely." If it is "merely" a psychological experience, it is nevertheless one of the utmost consequence. It makes all the difference between a life with or without creative meaning. "If you sum up what people tell you about their experience, you can formulate it about in this way: They came to themselves, they could accept themselves, they were able to become reconciled to themselves and by this they were also reconciled to adverse circumstances and events. This is much like what was formerly expressed by saying: He has made his peace with God, he has sacrificed his own will, he has submitted himself to the will of God."[8] They have experienced themselves as "the object of an unknown and superordinated subject," that is of the self which is "the most complete expression of that fateful combination we call individuality," and which is therefore "also the goal

---

[1] Jung, *Psychologie und Alchemie*, p. 28.
[2] Ibid., p. 35.
[8] Jung, *Psychology and Religion*, p. 99.

of life.''[1] It is in this sense that Jung has said that nobody is really cured "who did not regain his religious outlook."[2]

This regained "religious outlook" is a fundamentally new step in human consciousness. It is no longer undoubting belief and blind faith—it is an individual and primordial experience. The crisis in religious faith has been created by the very fact that man's growing individuality could no longer accept the traditional statements of faith as sufficiently convincing and binding. "He wants to break with tradition so that he can experiment with his life and determine what value and meaning things have in themselves, apart from traditional presuppositions."[3] This is not so much a deliberate act of rejection but rather an inner doubt which has forced itself on man as a consequence of an age-long process of individuation of human consciousness. As a matter of fact it is not only not deliberate but even dreaded and therefore often covered up. Nobody chooses willingly to be thrust out of the security and warmth of the motherly embrace—it is the progressive process of life that forces him to leave it.

In the "matriarchal" state of human consciousness, as it was expressed through the containment of man in the *"ecclesia mater,"* the inner psychic images of man had been more or less completely projected into external religious concepts and statements. "In an external form of religion, where the emphasis is completely on the external figure (in other words where a more or less complete projection exists), the archetype is identical with the external ideas, but remains unconscious as psychic

---

[1] Jung, *Two Essays on Analytical Psychology*, p. 268.
[2] Jung, *Modern Man in Search of a Soul*, p. 264.
[3] Ibid., p. 275f. Naturally, these statements are valid only for the highest level of present-day consciousness, i.e. for "the man of the immediate present." "Even in our civilizations the people who form, psychologically speaking, the lowest stratum, live almost as unconsciously as primitive races. Those of the succeeding stratum manifest a level of consciousness which corresponds to the beginnings of human culture, while those of the highest stratum have a consciousness capable of keeping step with the life of the last few centuries. Only the man who is modern in our meaning of the term really lives in the present; he alone has a present-day consciousness, and he alone finds that the ways of life which correspond to earlier levels pall upon him. . . ." (loc. cit., p. 227f.)

factor. If an unconscious content is in this way represented as a projected image it cannot become alive in the conscious mind or influence it. This means that it loses its creative life to a large extent."[1]

This explains why, with growing consciousness, man no longer found his creative impulses expressed in the images of religion. His new state of consciousness asked for something more than faith—it asked for experience. For a considerable time this need of experience was expressed by and lived out in the experience of external nature. When, however, man once more became aware of the question of the meaning of his life, his insistence on and his sharpened sense for individual experience could provide him with quite a new possibility. He turned his scientific enquiries on to his own inner condition—just as for a long time he had turned them on to his external situation. In his own empirical and experimental enquiry he was now able to discover the inner images—the archetypes—full of numinous significance. What had formerly been projected into external systems of faith—and had therefore been unconscious as a psychic factor—could thus become an internal experience which could be integrated into an enlarged consciousness. If the divine image can no longer be projected, the psychic energy invested in it is withdrawn and is bound to activate the corresponding psychic experience, the self or the "homo totus."[2]

The clash of the two conflicting powers—of the feminine, traditional, passive attitude that goes with an unconscious relatedness to the image of "wholeness," and of the masculine, enquiring, active one that goes with the loss of this relatedness but also with heightened consciousness—has produced its synthesis out of itself. This is the experience of the archetype of the "self," "which—as union of the opposites—mediates between the unconscious foundations and the conscious mind. It builds a bridge between modern consciousness which is menaced by alienation from its roots and the natural unconscious whole-

[1] Jung, *Psychologie und Alchemie*, p. 23.
[2] Cf. Jung, *Psychology and Religion*, pp. 105f.

ness of a more primitive age which is near to the instincts."[1] In other words: the "feminine" and "masculine" psychic factors, the unconscious and the conscious poles of the personality, are united in a psychic totality to which—to use the language of alchemy—one could also apply the symbol of the "hermaphrodite" or "rebis."[2] As it is the synthesis between the masculine and feminine elements—between "hermetic" gold and silver—alchemy uses also the image of the child, the *"filius philosophorum"* which is also the symbol for the philosopher's stone. As a matter of fact, this symbol of the child occurs frequently in unconscious clinical material as symbol of the self.[3]

It is interesting to notice in this connection how these unconscious contents first became conscious in projections. When, in particular since the French Enlightenment, the ego, that is the conscious mind, had become more and more identified with the whole personality, the unconscious, in its personification as woman, reasserted itself in an indirect way: Woman became more and more emancipated. (Similarly, with the loss of the uniting symbol, the interest in pedagogics became stimulated to such a degree that our century has even been called "the century of the child.")

The emancipation of woman is of the greatest psychological significance. Through it man has been presented in a concrete form with the problem of the feminine side of life. He has been obliged to acknowledge the existence of an autonomous and independent feminine psyche. His old-established belief in the "superiority" of the "logos" has been decisively challenged by the equally important, but diligently overlooked power of the

---

[1] Jung, *Das Göttliche Kind*, p. 116.

[2] Cf. Jung, *The Integration of the Personality*, p. 189 *et passim*. Jung had become interested in the hermetic side of alchemy, because patients produced dreams containing alchemical symbols. Thus Jung discovered that alchemy is a symbolical representation of the individuation process. In this sense alchemy is a pre-stage of the modern psychology of the unconscious. As to the "lapis," the rebis or hermaphrodite, Jung remarks: "All these symbols in the last analysis depicted this state of affairs that we call the self, in its rôle of transcending consciousness." (loc. cit.)

[3] As to the symbolism of the child cf. in particular Jung's *Das Göttliche Kind*.

"eros."[1] Where this challenge is accepted and answered in a constructive sense, a new and creative relationship between man and woman as equal partners can be established. Here the inner process of the synthesis between the feminine and the masculine psyche, of the creation of the total personality, has found its concrete externalized expression.

As long as it remains only an external event—even though a most creative one—it has not fully fulfilled itself. The self is the *whole* of man, that is, it represents the complete relation between the outside and the inside. Thus in the experience of the self the synthesis between the feminine and the masculine principles is lived in both aspects, as individual and creative relationship between man and woman outside, and between masculine and feminine psychic contents inside. The two experiences go hand in hand, and thus the inner realization of the "conjunctio," of the "union of the opposites" *in* man leads finally to the fully integrated and individuated personality. This process, however few may be aware of it or irresistibly seized by its inner logic, is on its way. With it modern man has been given his highest chance: the reconciliation of a conflict which for centuries has been his psychic wound. C. G. Jung has played a part in the reconciliation of this conflict which, we hope, will yet prove of the utmost consequence. He has given modern man just those tools and realizations which he needs to bridge the gap between his ego and his soul.

"Analysis is always followed by synthesis, and what had been separated on a deeper level is always reunited on a higher one."[2]

1Cf. Jung's essay, "Woman in Europe," in *Contributions to Analytical Psychology*.
2Jung, *Paracelsica*, p. 178.

INDEX